About the Author

Sarah Napthali is the author of the international bestseller *Buddhism for Mothers*, which has been translated into 13 languages and sold over 100,000 copies. Sarah wrote a further four books about applying Buddhist teachings in family life, including *Buddhism for Mothers of Young Children*, *Buddhism for Mothers of School Children*, *Buddhism for Parents on the Go*, and *Buddhism for Couples*. She lives in Sydney, not too far from her two adult sons.

MY YEAR OF PSYCHEDELICS

Exploring the amazing potential of mushrooms, MDMA, LSD and other life-enhancing substances

SARAH NAPTHALI

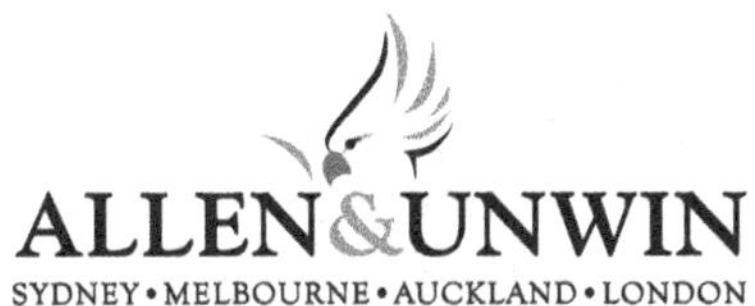

First published in 2025

Some names and identifying details have been changed to protect the privacy of individuals.

Allen & Unwin
Cammeraygal Country
83 Alexander Street
Crows Nest NSW 2065
Australia
Phone: (61 2) 8425 0100
Email: info@allenandunwin.com
Web: www.allenandunwin.com

Allen & Unwin acknowledges the Traditional Owners of the Country on which we live and work. We pay our respects to all Aboriginal and Torres Strait Islander Elders, past and present.

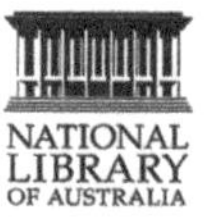

A catalogue record for this book is available from the National Library of Australia

ISBN 978 1 76147 062 2

p. 2: Grateful acknowledgement is given for permission to reprint 'The Most Dangerous Drugs' from Nutt, King & Phillips, 'Drug harms in the UK: a multicriteria decision analysis, *The Lancet*, Volume. 376, Issue 9752 (2010), pp. 1558–1565.

Set in 12.25/18.5 pt Adobe Garamond Pro by Bookhouse, Sydney

10 9 8 7 6 5 4 3 2 1

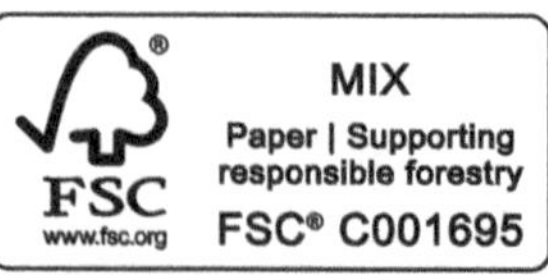

MY YEAR OF PSYCHEDELICS

Exploring the amazing potential of mushrooms, MDMA, LSD and other life-enhancing substances

SARAH NAPTHALI

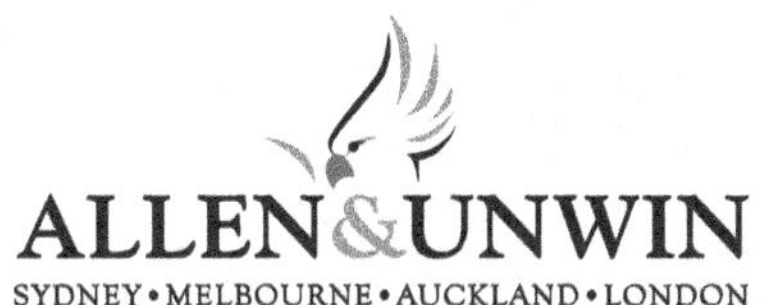

First published in 2025

Some names and identifying details have been changed to protect the privacy of individuals.

Allen & Unwin
Cammeraygal Country
83 Alexander Street
Crows Nest NSW 2065
Australia
Phone: (61 2) 8425 0100
Email: info@allenandunwin.com
Web: www.allenandunwin.com

Allen & Unwin acknowledges the Traditional Owners of the Country on which we live and work. We pay our respects to all Aboriginal and Torres Strait Islander Elders, past and present.

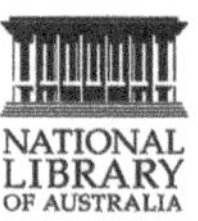

A catalogue record for this book is available from the National Library of Australia

ISBN 978 1 76147 062 2

p. 2: Grateful acknowledgement is given for permission to reprint 'The Most Dangerous Drugs' from Nutt, King & Phillips, 'Drug harms in the UK: a multicriteria decision analysis, *The Lancet*, Volume. 376, Issue 9752 (2010), pp. 1558–1565.

Set in 12.25/18.5 pt Adobe Garamond Pro by Bookhouse, Sydney

10 9 8 7 6 5 4 3 2 1

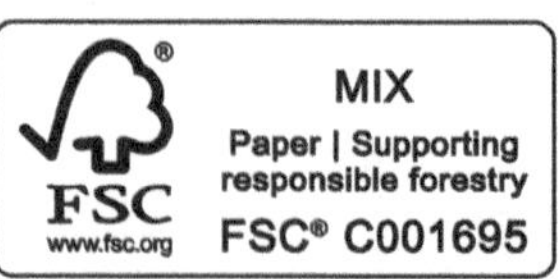

The paper in this book is FSC® certified. FSC® promotes environmentally responsible, socially beneficial and economically viable management of the world's forests.

Contents

This book does not promote taking illicit substances. Time has shown that people will take psychoactive substances, legal or not. As such, this book seeks to promote harm minimisation by exploring safe approaches.

Introduction

Confession: I've always been fascinated by illegal drugs.

That's not to say I spent my youth indulging. I didn't. My experience is quite negligible.

It's more a matter that, over decades, I've read many books on the subject, listened to a string of podcasts and picked any drug user's brain about their experiences. I even trained and became a volunteer for a telephone support service for family members affected by substance use. With a monthly shift for over four years, I became well aware of the damage illicit drugs can do to both users and their families. Yet it would be unrealistic to paint all drugs with the same brush for, as with legal drugs, some can be dangerous for certain people, while some can enhance our lives.

Maybe the seed of this decades-long curiosity was planted on my commute to high school by the overlarge graffiti in the train tunnel at St Leonards:

REALITY IS FOR PEOPLE WHO CAN'T HANDLE DRUGS.

I pondered this daily as a schoolgirl—although I never took action. I never moved in the kind of crowd that had the access to, or inclination for, recreational drug use. Yet I always remained curious to experience 'altered states of consciousness'. I didn't want to reach the end of my life having missed opportunities to expand my mind, to benefit from epiphanies, great highs and deep insights. I always wanted to avoid any semblance of sleepwalking through my days in the trance of habits and routines, stagnating. I wanted a showdown with the bogeymen lurking in my unconscious mind who obstruct my capacity to live my happiest life.

I guess I have a personality type that wants to experience everything and never, never miss out. In my youth, I assumed travel would fulfil this desire—if I could just travel to enough countries, experience some different cultures, then I'd be a complete person. This assumption eventually morphed into the belief that if I met enough people, from a wide range of life experiences, then I'd have a grip on what life is all about. That belief became: if I could just read enough books and increase my general knowledge, about philosophy, psychology and spirituality, then that might make me whole. My patchwork of a résumé suggests I applied this thinking to jobs, too, as I kept trying out new ones rather than staying anywhere for more than a few years. All of which brought me to now, where I flirt with the idea that if I could imbibe some mind-expanding substances, I could learn about what else there is and dramatically broaden my understanding of how to be the wisest human I could be.

On my 55th birthday, I made a promise that I'd find safe ways to provide myself with the very experiences that could open 'the doors of perception', as author Aldous Huxley named his classic book about his foray into the psychedelic drug mescaline. My marriage had ended, the kids had left home, I'd downsized to a smaller house and dropped down to four days of work—now was the time. I stood before the window between the years of responsibility behind me and the health problems of old age. I would learn firsthand what was meant by phrases such as 'ego death', 'oneness with everything', 'transcendence'.

Of course, I wouldn't go near any dangerous drugs like methamphetamine or prescription opiates. Rather, I'd experiment with a class of drugs where addiction, let alone an overdose or death, would not be an issue. Low in toxicity, low in their potential for abuse, psychedelics—magic mushrooms, ayahuasca and LSD—would be my drugs of choice. In fact, I'd have to stop using the word 'drugs', as I'd soon discover that most in the psychedelic world refer to psychedelics as 'medicines'.

My meditation practice had definitely helped me to be calmer, more patient and loving. It allowed me to increase my self-awareness and better regulate the tumultuous emotions of the Highly Sensitive Person that I am. Yet I never had the powers of concentration that would allow for the great spiritual awakenings we hear of: the dissolution of the Self, the loss of feelings of separation from others, or insights into the true nature of reality. Perhaps an even larger question was why, in my fifties, was I still plagued with self-doubt, moodiness and impatience? What I needed was a faster-acting mechanism for change than my meditation skills could provide.

The word psychedelic is made up of 'psyche' meaning mind and 'delic' meaning reveal. What I envisioned was a journey revealing the secrets hidden in my own mind. I'd heard, more than once, claims similar to those found in a 2006 study in which a staggering 67 per cent of the 24 volunteers rated their experience with psilocybin to be either the single most meaningful experience of their life or among the top five.[1] Similarly, Steve Jobs claimed that 'doing LSD was one of the two or three most important things I have done in my life'.[2] Perhaps we should see a psychedelic experience as a birthright that successive governments around the world have denied us?

Psychedelics are a class of psychoactive substances that produce changes in perception and mood. They affect all the senses, and alter our thinking, sense of time and emotions. They can cause us to hallucinate—to see or hear things that might not exist or are distorted. I've heard of dramatic emotional breakthroughs and spiritual realisations.

Aren't you a bit old for this? is one obvious question. On the contrary, as renowned author Michael Pollan writes, psychedelics are 'wasted on the young'.[3] Pollan appeared on the list of *Time Magazine*'s Top 100 Most Influential People in the World back in 2010 having written several books about plants with a focus on nutrition. His book on psychedelics, *How To Change Your Mind: The new science of psychedelics*, published in 2018, opened my eyes to the immense potential of which I'd been ignorant. Pollan argues that it's older people who could benefit the most from psychedelics as the middle-aged are more likely to be stuck in their ways, or rigid in their thinking. This struck a powerful chord with me as I could see certain aspects of my life becoming somewhat 'set': the fixed way I perceived certain relationships, my knee-jerk reactions to stressors and irritations, my preoccupation with working through the to-do list as though nothing else mattered.

Pollan has been a boon to the world of psychedelics in that he is a science writer in his sixties, a family man who is anything but a hippie, a dropout, a misfit or any of the labels traditionally attributed to the stereotype of those who use psychedelics. Pollan has been instrumental in assisting psychedelics to lose their image as drugs for those on the fringe. I'm a tax-paying, fully vaxxed, pro-recycling, middle-aged mother, yet I'm keen to follow his lead and discover what psychedelics can do for me.

Pollan uses a beautiful metaphor, borrowed from a Dutch neuroscientist, where he asks us to imagine our thoughts are sleds travelling down a snowy mountain. The more the sleds travel down, the deeper the grooves, until eventually there is no choice but to fall into those grooves. So too, older people potentially start to follow a predetermined script with default reactions to every situation. Pollan's neuroscientist argues that psychedelics are like having a new snowfall that covers up all those grooves, giving us a fresh start.

As attractive as this metaphor is, I can't help questioning how true it could be. Surely, if rewriting all our thoughts and habits was as simple as taking a psychedelic, wouldn't everyone be doing exactly that, legal or not? How miraculous could these substances really be? Would they be a panacea, or just a handy part of a larger toolkit? Either way, I was determined to find out for myself.

Our culture has come to associate psychedelics with youth, parties and law-breaking. Yet the foremost expert on mushrooms in the world, mycologist Paul Stamets, argues that mushrooms need to be taken seriously for not only their medicinal value but for the life-changing spiritual experiences they can provide. He should know: they cured him of stuttering when he was a teenager. He abhors the frivolous slang 'shrooms'.[4]

I was satisfied that age was no barrier to taking psychedelics, but there was still the not insignificant question of the law. In Australia, the so-called war on drugs sees policy makers label all drugs as dangerous. Alas, my only option, at least initially, was to travel to countries where professional health workers, or experienced shamans and guides, run psychedelic retreats for groups. This was the perfect option for a Nervous Nellie like me—supervised ceremonies with plenty of focus on safety and the creation of the best conditions possible. On such retreats, the drugs are incorporated into programs of anything from three to ten days that involve the three steps of: 1) preparation, 2) ceremony, and 3) integration. The focus would be on relaxing in the lead-up to the ceremony—through yoga, meditation, good nutrition, group discussions—before taking the drug as part of a united community. Integration afterwards, for the mind and body, would be key to making any new discoveries stick. Such conditions are seen as sound insurance against a 'bad' trip. At least, I'd be able to do a retreat for three of the eight medicines I wanted to try.

I won't lie: I had my reservations about this project. I'm not at an age where I take mental or physical health lightly. With my hypochondriac tendencies I spend my days preoccupied by concepts like 'prevention', 'nutrition', 'physical and mental fitness' and meticulous 'self-care'. For months I finished my day lying in bed sleepless, gripped with myriad fears. Does this project mean sacrificing my precious body to research? What if I have a bad trip? I've heard bad trips can last for hours, or seem to. What if I have a psychotic episode from which I never recover? Far from home, in a foreign land. I'd heard that vomiting was inevitable after taking the Amazonian medicine ayahuasca. I hate vomiting more than anything.

Would dabbling with psychedelics affect my sleep—the most important element of my wellbeing? Then there was the fact that I'm a sensitive unit. I have a small build and can easily feel ill after small amounts of alcohol, caffeine, sugar or rich food. I feel slightly high after a cup of tea. Not joking.

How would this project affect Luke, my new partner of one year? I adore him and don't want to lose him by behaving like a loose cannon full of whacky ideas. He's too wary to try any psychedelics himself, despite being a most happy drinker. How would he feel about me tripping my way around the world?

Evidence for a psychedelic renaissance abounds. Take Netflix. The number of documentaries suggests something big is afoot. There's the docuseries *How To Change Your Mind* based on Michael Pollan's book of the same name. There's the first episode of Gwyneth Paltrow's *Goop Lab* where her team go on a mushroom, or psilocybin, retreat. Other shows include *Fantastic Fungi* featuring interviews with mycologist Paul Stamets and author Michael Pollan; and *Have a Good Trip: Adventures in Psychedelics* in which a stream of celebrities, including Sting, describe their psychedelic experiences. Then there are a gazillion podcasts about psychedelics by the likes of the most popular podcaster in the world, Joe Rogan, or investor

Tim Ferriss, who's donated over 2 million dollars of his own funds to psychedelic research.[5]

Perhaps the most exciting finding about psychedelics is what happens in the days *after* you take them, for neuroscientists have discovered that psychedelics create a window of 'neuroplasticity', a period where new connections are made allowing for changes in neural networks.[6] This happens because a part of the brain called the 'default mode network', where all the forms of self-focus occur—such as worry, rumination or daydreaming—starts to go quiet, or as scientists put it 'down-regulate'. When the default mode network is less active, new connections form between parts of the brain that never used to talk to each other.

Brain imaging reveals that the brain on psychedelics resembles the brain of an experienced meditator.[7] It also reveals that the experience of ego dissolution, where the sense of a separate self disappears, is common to both experienced meditators and the brain on psychedelics and coincides with low activity in the default mode network. Sadly, I'm an experienced meditator with no experience of ego dissolution, probably because it's exceedingly difficult, if not impossible, to quieten my particular mind for any long stretch of time.

For those who'd like a trip without the legal risks, or the expense of travelling to a country where it's legal, there's holotropic breathwork, invented in the 1970s and investigated in Chapter 9. Good news for many, breath exercises can induce a non-ordinary state of consciousness similar to, if not as intense as, a psychedelic experience.

I've found that even reading about psychedelics changes the quality of my daily state of consciousness. Informed about other mind-states, I find myself more open to awe and wonder as I walk down the streets I see every day. I'm more present, more open to my surroundings and how miraculous they are. The mere existence of psychedelics reminds us that there are more ways to be conscious than our daily habitual state has to offer, which for most of us can be described as 'lost in our heads' or lost in thoughts of the past and future.

Inspired by Michael Pollan, I tried a psychedelic in recent years. I'd read his book *How To Change Your Mind* in 2018 and became determined to have my own psychedelic experience. Pollan had tracked down every expert in the field before plunging in, despite his nerves, to try a range of different psychedelics. He experienced an array of epiphanies and spiritual peaks that I had never even come close to through my meditation practice with my weak powers of concentration. His experiences with psychedelics led him to start a meditation practice, something he told podcaster Dan Harris that he'd never considered previously.[8]

For many months I put out the word that I was looking for mushrooms and I kept my eyes peeled on bushwalks after rain. My son Zac had assured me, 'They're everywhere'. Zac was wrong. Eventually he took me to a spot by a river, five minutes' drive from my home, where I picked my first mushrooms. Zac showed me that when he squeezed the stem, it turned a shade of blue, indicating the presence of psilocybin. He was also able to reassure me that he knew a few locals who had eaten from this location and come to no harm. My second-born, Alex, now a grown-up (of sorts), agreed to be with me for the ingestion. I munched them down lying on the couch in my living room and waited for something to happen. Soon enough Alex's phone rang. His friends wanted him to join them, to which he replied, 'Sorry, I'm trip-sitting my mum.' My God, what was I doing?

Of course, one advantage of sharing the details of a psychedelic journey with your adult children is that it opens up a conversation about safety. When they are free to speak openly about their own psychedelic use, you can pursue harm reduction and encourage them, for example, to use pill-testing kits, which are cheap and easy to purchase online.

The mushrooms made me feel wobbly and pleasantly drunk. I lay on the couch and enjoyed what Zac called 'visuals'—images that appear in the mind's eye, usually brightly coloured moving patterns, although they weren't particularly amazing. Except for one image where I gazed up, at a forest from among the roots of a tree as though from a worm's perspective. For a fleeting moment I felt a beautiful feeling of peace and a sense that nature, its beauty and perfection, will always be there for me, to provide reassurance and comfort. Other than a few moments that have stayed with me strongly, the experience, overall, was underwhelming. For a couple of hours I felt a lethargy that was similar to suffering a heavy cold.

I moaned to Zac, who moved in and out of the room, 'I don't have any energy. I just feel restless.'

'Surrender to it, Mum,' he told me. 'You don't always have to rush around.'

Nup, I thought over the following days. I like to feel motivated and energised. None of this zonked-out state for me. In retrospect, taking psychedelics in my home was the wrong setting as I associate home, sadly enough, with busyness and 'getting things done'. I gave up on psychedelics and didn't think about them again until about three years later, when I started watching Michael Pollan's docuseries on Netflix and I became obsessed all over again. *I need to do this properly*, I thought. *I'm going to experience the real deal, whatever it takes.*

There was one more problem to solve concerning my psychedelic project. I would need to attend retreats in both Europe and South America. I was confident to travel alone in Europe, a place I was familiar with after twenty years married to a European with whom I'd visited several countries on the continent, but how could I go to South America on my own? For an ayahuasca retreat, South America would be my destination as the plant grows in the Amazon jungle. For the last five years, my job has been supporting victims of sexual assault, and other crimes, as they endure the trials of the criminal justice system. This work makes me hypervigilant about my personal safety: I would be a small woman with only a smattering of Spanish—I needed a travel companion. Moreover, any anxiety about my personal safety could spill into my psychedelic experiences, at worst, leading to 'bad' trips. I knew it was important to come to psychedelics with a calm mind to ensure the best experience. My partner Luke wouldn't attend a retreat, but he promised to accompany me to South America for a holiday.

My odyssey could begin.

I

Isn't it all a bit risky?

For the overwhelming majority of people, my research suggests, psychedelics, used in the right setting and with a calm mindset, are safe. That said, psychedelic retreats screen participants to exclude those vulnerable to psychosis. Psychedelics can apparently cause long-term mental health issues in patients with a predisposition to bipolar disorder or schizophrenia. Such disorders are more likely to be provoked in the young, rather than the middle-aged, given that those diagnoses tend to emerge in one's twenties.

The following graph says it all. Alcohol, which few question, is far more dangerous, to individuals and to society, than psychedelic drugs. The graph was prepared by the Independent Scientific Committee on Drugs in the UK and measures both dangers to the user and to others.[1] It ranked twenty drugs on sixteen measures of harm, after scoring each drug for mental and physical damage, addiction, crime and costs to the economy and communities. It found ecstasy (the street name for MDMA) and LSD were among the least damaging, with mushrooms at the very bottom of the list.

The most dangerous drugs

Ranked by drug experts on damage to user, impact on crime, and socioeconomic effects

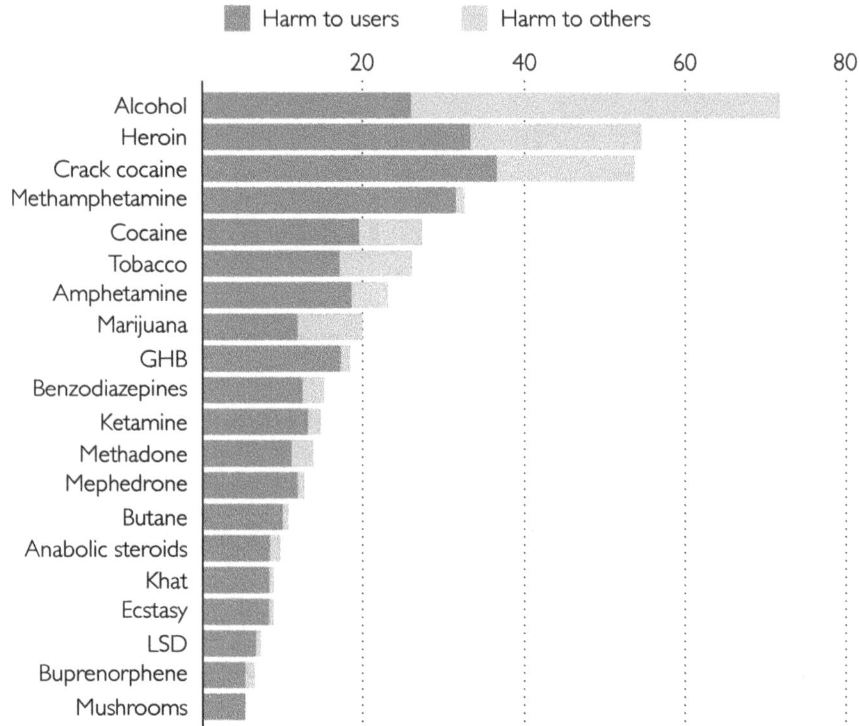

Source: Independent Scientific Committee on Drugs, based on analysis of UK drug use, *The Lancet*, 2010

I listened to a Joe Rogan podcast where he interviewed Rick Doblin, the founder of MAPS, a research and educational body making excellent progress in the push to legalise MDMA and other psychedelics to treat mental illness. Doblin explained that for any drug to be safe, it needs to be used for the right purpose and in

the right way because 'they're just tools'. He gave thalidomide as an example: it was the wrong tool to treat morning sickness and caused deformities in babies, but today, thalidomide is an effective medicine for treating cancers and leprosies. Rogan clarified: 'I give you a hammer. You could build a house, or you could hit yourself in the dick.'[2]

In the interests of balance, I'll include a quotation from *The Psychedelic Explorer's Guide* by Jim Fadiman, a book that many retreat centres advise visitors to read before attending. The book is, as one would guess, consistently enthusiastic about psychedelics and their potential—except for this paragraph:

> Even the most pro-psychedelic advocate needs to keep in mind that these substances, when misused and even used with care, have caused serious and lasting mental damage.[3]

That was a shock. Would I be the one? Should I cancel the whole project before it's too late? Then I remembered reading a similar cautionary tale about attending mindfulness retreats. It's not unheard of for a person to leave a mindfulness retreat with ongoing mental illness[4]—I've never met anyone this happened to during all the years I've spent in Buddhist circles, but I've read about it. I concluded that any activity in life presents some danger, not least, the activities we engage in as part of ordinary life, such as driving, drinking alcohol, having babies or playing sports. Yet most of us continue to engage in such pursuits despite the risks. I remained satisfied, from the vast amount of information I'd absorbed from books, podcasts and discussions, that the risk of developing a mental illness was too small for me to worry about.

Leading neuropsychopharmacologist Professor David Nutt supports my conclusion. In his recently published book *Psychedelics: The revolutionary drugs that could change your life—a guide from the expert*, he wrote of psychedelics: 'They have risks and side effects, as do all medicines, and it's true that people have died or suffered after taking these substances; but, most of the risk of taking them comes from them being illicit and how and where illicit drugs are taken.'[5] Their illicit status, he explains, leads to dangers like contamination, ignorance about dosage, use by people prone to psychosis who should avoid them, or use with the wrong mindset or in an inappropriate setting.

Nutt cites a study of 130,000 people comparing the mental health of those who have taken psychedelics with those who haven't. Of that large sample, 13 per cent of them had taken psychedelics and the researchers found: '. . . those people were no more likely than those who hadn't to have had recent anxiety, depression, suicidality or any other serious psychological distress and . . . in several cases psychedelic use was associated with lower rates of mental health problems.' He mentions another study comparing the mental health of those who had and hadn't taken psychedelics, a study of over 190,000 people, that found 'having used psychedelics was associated with a reduced likelihood of psychological distress in the past month, and of suicidality in the past year'.

Researchers in the field all concede that ongoing negative effects on mental health can happen, but they settle on the word 'rare' to describe the frequency.

Not only has the war on drugs exaggerated the risk posed by psychedelics to our mental health but it has also established the idea in the collective mind that they are addictive. My son Zac was the first to dispel this myth for me when he said, 'A high-dose psychedelic experience is so dramatic that you won't be ready to go back for more for a few months. It's too exhausting,' and that would not be the last time I heard this sentiment.

Professor Nutt also dispels most worries about addictiveness:

> Treatment facilities aren't full of people who are dependent on LSD or psilocybin. The key to this is their effect on the brain. Psychedelics do produce a very rapid desensitisation or tolerance response. Keep taking LSD and the euphoric and psychedelic effects quickly decrease. However, unlike addictive drugs, taking more does not bring the effects back, i.e., even if you wanted more of the effects (and not everyone does), you couldn't get them.

As with any negative effects on mental health, addiction, too, is possible and is probably more likely for MDMA than for the other medicines I intended to try, but once more, the word I found again and again in the research, when it came to addiction, was 'rare'.

Many users, few addicts

Well over a decade ago, I attended a weekend of training to become a telephone volunteer on a support line. Family Drug Support was founded by Tony Trimingham, author of *Not My Family, Never My Child*, who lost his 23-year-old son Damien to a heroin overdose in 1997.[6] The experience prompted him to offer to the families of drug users the support he wishes he'd had.[7] Once a month for four years, I'd work a four-hour shift speaking to family members, mainly parents, about the challenges they faced when a family member's substance use became problematic. The moment that stood out for me on the first day of training was when Tony told us that 80 to 90 per cent of users of any drug will not become addicted. I stopped breathing for a few moments to process this. Could that be true? My father had told me from a young age that if I so much as tried marijuana, the 'gateway drug', there would be a natural progression through all the different drugs until I arrived at heroin—and died. Of course, I no longer believed this but some of the message was, clearly, still in my DNA.

I decided to check more recent figures. One literature review began thus:

> . . . the majority of drug use is episodic, transient and generally non-problematic. The majority of people who have used various drugs in their lifetime have not done so in the past year. Only a minority become problem drug users.[8]

The review offered the figure of 11.6 per cent; that is to say: 11.6 per cent of all the illegal drug users in the world suffered problematic drug use or addiction. *Who are this 11.6 per cent?* anxious parents ask themselves. My time fielding phone calls for Family Drug Support left me with the impression that those in trouble had pre-existing underlying vulnerabilities. I can't remember a call where problematic drug use was only about the drug and no other variables. It was more likely to be about a combination of variables, such as a mental health diagnosis, past trauma, unemployment, chronic isolation or just a tough period of life to navigate.

Paul Hayes would agree. He's an honorary professor of drug policy at the London School of Hygiene and Tropical Medicine and the former CEO of the National Treatment Agency for Substance Misuse where he was responsible to the UK Parliament for the delivery of treatment for drug addiction in England between 2001 and 2013. He wrote an article for online journal *The Conversation*,[9] where all articles are written by academics with support from journalists, entitled 'Many people use drugs—but here's why most don't become addicts'. He claims that the majority of drug users are 'intelligent resourceful people with good life skills, supportive networks and loving families'. They have structures in place, such as family support, a job and prospects for the future, that all serve to protect them from problematic use. Hayes describes what it's like for those who lack these supports:

> In contrast the most vulnerable individuals in our poorest communities lack life skills and have networks that entrench their problems rather than offering solutions. Their decision making will tend to prioritise immediate benefit rather than long-term consequences. The multiplicity of overlapping challenges they face gives them little incentive to avoid high risk behaviours . . . instead of carefully calibrating their drug use to minimise risk, they will be prepared to use the most dangerous drugs in the most dangerous ways. And once addicted, motivation to recover and the likelihood of success is weakened by an absence of family support, poor prospects of employment, insecure housing and social isolation.

Even if the risk of addiction has been exaggerated in the rhetoric of the war on drugs, other risks are worth taking seriously. The most significant health risk is that due to the illegality of psychedelic substances, pills such as MDMA are sometimes only accessible through those greedy and reckless enough to provide a contaminated product. This risk can be mitigated by ordering a drug testing kit online, which is not expensive. It's a shame, ridiculous even, that most state and territory governments in Australia have not approved pill testing at music festivals, which could save young lives.[10]

Go ask Alice

What had made me assume, for all those years before the Family Drug Support training, that all illicit drugs were incredibly dangerous? I know that one contributor was a book that everyone at my school had read called *Go Ask Alice,* by the intriguing 'Anonymous'.[11] Published in 1971, this 'diary' of a fifteen-year-old girl from the US was accepted as proof that one could move from marijuana to heroin in a short amount of time. Alice's first exposure to drugs was at a party when someone spiked her soda with LSD; then, within a week she was on the drug speed. From there it was a slippery slope to homelessness, sex work and eventual overdose, the epilogue reading: 'The subject of this book died three weeks after her decision not to keep another diary. Her parents came home from a movie and found her dead. They called the police and the hospital but there was nothing anyone could do.'

Excuse the above spoiler, but the book isn't worth reading. Other dramatic diary entries included: 'Today I sold ten stamps of LSD to a little kid at the grade school who was not even nine years old.'

And: 'Another day, another blow job.'

With sales well over 5 million, the book has never been out of print; it became a high-rating TV movie and a play, and won numerous awards. Yet author Rick Emerson revealed the diary to be a hoax in his book *Unmask Alice: LSD, satanic panic, and the imposter behind the world's most notorious diaries,* as he found no evidence over his seven years of research that the teenager existed.[12] It seems she was a figment of the imagination of the late author Beatrice Sparks, who had a track record in publishing fake teen diaries albeit loosely based on real people. Alice may have been vaguely similar to a troubled young girl Beatrice had met in her volunteer role as a youth counsellor.

How could we all have been tricked like this? How did this even happen? Emerson explains that *Go Ask Alice* was born when twenty-year-old Diane Linkletter jumped from the window of her Los Angeles apartment. Her father, Art Linkletter, had been a famous TV personality, a household name. Linkletter was understandably desperate for answers as to why his daughter would jump to her death. He blamed LSD, which she'd taken six months prior. The toxicology report then revealed the absence of any drugs, so he blamed an 'LSD flashback'. President Nixon soon invited him to the White House, recognising that he might be a perfect weapon for his war on drugs. The media fanned the flames, providing endless coverage of this LSD-induced suicide with headlines like 'LSD killed Diane.'

Enter Beatrice Sparks, who had at one point worked with Linkletter on a failed publishing project. When she showed Linkletter a collection of diary pages he immediately found her a publisher.

What about lingering effects?

One man for whom psychedelics have caused a fair degree of suffering is Englishman Jules Evans. After taking psychedelics as a teenager, in less-than-ideal settings, he suffered years of PTSD and social anxiety. Twenty years later, feeling more psychologically robust, he decided to give them another try and attended an ayahuasca retreat in Peru. He enjoyed the retreat, and gained many valuable insights, however, as soon as the retreat was over, he experienced what many call a 'spiritual emergency': he suffered a period of fear and disorientation that lasted two weeks.[13] Today, he heads the Challenging Psychedelic Experiences Project where a team researches difficulties caused by psychedelics and what helps people deal with them.[14]

His team surveyed a sample of 608 people who had experienced 'extended difficulties after using psychedelics' and found:

> . . . one third reported difficulties lasting longer than a year and one sixth longer than three years. The most common reported difficulties were anxiety, social disconnection, derealization, existential struggle and continued visual distortions. And 8% of survey respondents had taken psychedelics in a therapeutic or clinical setting, so harms happen even under 'safe' settings.

Jules's voice, and the project itself, is important in the psychedelic space, to put the brakes on any hype, provide a mechanism to hold the facilitators of the psychedelic renaissance to account and to remind us all to be cautious—the medicines are powerful.

What about 'bad trips'?

Buddhist teachers say there is no such thing as a 'bad' meditation session—even if our attention is scattered, we at least cultivate awareness of our scattered state of mind. Moreover, perhaps the thoughts that arise are important ones that we need to address. The same can be said for 'bad' psychedelic trips. The singer Sting said in the documentary *Have a Good Trip*, 'Whenever I've had a bad trip—and I've had many—I always realise that it was what I needed. Sometimes it kicks your arse and sometimes you need to have your ego taken down a notch or two.' He went on to talk about the positive experiences 'of love, support, a sense of buoyancy, a religious sense of connection to the planet' concluding with the words, 'my feeling is it balances out'.

The accepted wisdom is that a difficult trip can sometimes be a gift, an opportunity to learn about our shadow side, or about how our unconscious mind holds us back. Another interpretation of a 'bad' trip is that it may be the result of 'resistance' or trying to stop whatever is arising, and occurs when we refuse to surrender to the experience.

Dying of curiosity, I was ready to surrender.

2

Lead-up to my first retreat

ONCE I'D MADE UP my mind to go to the Netherlands for a psilocybin retreat—psilocybin being the psychoactive part of magic mushrooms—it was quite an undertaking to google all the retreats as there was no lack of them, only a lack of retreats that were not already booked out. I was anxious about a budget blowout from my project, so I settled on a short three-day retreat run by an organisation called the Essence Institute. They ran several retreats a month, but I kept missing out—they sold out fast and, before I knew it, they were booked out for months in advance. The psychedelic renaissance was real.

My partner Luke was a useful devil's advocate as I sifted through the options.

'Who's running these retreats? How do you know they're not charlatans? Can you trust them?'

'I'm not worried,' I replied. 'The people running them are mental health professionals—psychologists, nurses or people with science degrees who have done courses in different therapies.'

Then I stumbled on a website called 'Awaken the Medicine Within'. The woman leading this retreat was Natasja Pelgrom. My research revealed that Natasja was a revered thought leader and had a background as an accomplished executive. In 2017, she launched the first women-led legal psychedelic retreat business in the European Union. Since then, she'd mentored many executives and organisations in the psychedelic space. She'd been an adviser to psychedelic researchers and had played pivotal roles in over 800 psychedelic ceremonies, where she'd served as a trainer, assistant and facilitator. It made sense to do a retreat with a woman informed by Western approaches such as neuroscience, but also by the indigenous peoples who'd been using the plants for millennia. Natasja seemed knowledgeable of the sacred rituals and numerous other elements required to provide a 'safe container' for a plant medicine experience.

This five-day retreat would cost double the shorter retreat, but it would definitely provide ample preparation and integration and the chance for me to take psilocybin properly in two ceremonies. I emailed Natasja:

> Good morning Natasja,
>
> I'd be interested in attending your retreat but I'm wondering if I could attend at a discount? I'm hoping to write a book about several retreats I attend around the world so I'm trying to keep costs down if I possibly can. Hopefully,

> I could let Australians know about your work if my book is ever published?

Natasja wrote back:

> Let's have a chat via Zoom.

First Zoom with Natasja

My first one-to-one Zoom with Natasja contained several setbacks, albeit minor, for my writing project.

'The ideal approach may be to stay with one plant medicine and try it in a range of contexts over time,' she suggested. This did not exactly chime with my book idea of investigating eight medicines.

Then she said, 'It has to be said, Sarah, integrity in the psychedelic space is incredibly important while society is still learning about them. You need to respect the confidentiality of others on the retreat, no matter what they say to you at the time, about permission to share any details of their experience.'

'Oh, I agree whole-heartedly,' I assured her while, at the same time, lamenting that I generally prefer to write about other people rather than only about myself.

'On another matter,' I asked nervously, 'I see from your website there's a diet for the week prior and I'd need to suspend my use of CBD and THC for a few weeks. I'm kind of completely dependent on medical cannabis to fall asleep at night.'

'Would you be able to switch to melatonin in the week before?' Natasja asked.

'Probably, I guess,' I said resisting the urge to grimace.

I had one more question for Natasja: 'I heard you in a podcast say that 90 per cent of people who do your retreats were inspired after reading Michael Pollan's book, which came out in 2018. Is that true?' I was sure this had been some kind of inadvertent exaggeration, but Natasja replied: 'Yes, they've all read that book.'

It's worth reflecting on the name Natasja had chosen for her retreat business, 'Awaken the Medicine Within'. Such a title reminds us that the answers are not outside us, as we routinely assume, or even in the plant medicine. In the words of one psychonaut I met, 'You are the medicine.' Thirteenth-century Sufi mystic and poet Rumi offers several quotations to this effect:

> 'The inspiration you seek is already within you. Be silent and listen.'
>
> 'We are one. Everything in the universe is within you. Ask all from yourself.'
>
> 'Why are you so enchanted by this world, when a mine of gold lies within you?'
>
> 'You have within you more love than you could ever understand.'

I'm reminded of a joke an Indian man once told me: One day God asked a wise man, 'Is there somewhere I can go to get away from all these humans and their endless requests?'

The wise man replied, 'Yes, go inside each one of them. They'll never look there.'

There was more bad news on the sleep front, however, quite apart from the jetlag of travelling across the world and suspending my CBD and THC. I received an email providing the dates of six Zoom meetings: three prior to the retreat entitled 'preparation' meetings, and three after the retreat called 'integration' meetings. These meetings were an integral part of the experience, and I was looking forward to them, except all six would occur at 4 a.m. Sydney time.

As I complained to my sons about all the sleep loss ahead, Zac raised: 'I don't know why you don't just pick some mushrooms down the road for free like last time you tried them?'

'I want to do this properly this time, Zac, with supervision, with someone who understands dosages and who can access the best mushrooms for the job.'

'Why don't you just go to Amsterdam?' suggested Zac, 'and buy mushroom truffles from one of their smartshops—they're cheap and legal.'

It was true that Amsterdam is the home of several smartshops selling, legally, various strains of magic mushrooms and other plant-based substances and supplements.

'If taking mushrooms could be one of the most meaningful experiences of my life, I may as well invest in doing it in the best conditions available.'

'Whatever,' Zac replied, shaking his head at the extreme cautiousness of the middle-aged.

Preparation

Natasja encouraged us to prepare ourselves 'emotionally, mentally, physically and spiritually'. Emotionally, we were to discover what needed healing or releasing within us, perhaps using journalling, meditation or time reflecting in nature. Mentally, we needed to research psilocybin, read the books, surf the net, so we could engage in the ceremony well-informed and free of any doubts that might affect our mindset. We needed to be ready to completely surrender. Resistance while on psychedelics is futile; you can't disembark the moving train. We also needed to knock things off our to-do list that might weigh on us—perhaps, find ways to declutter our desks, houses and minds or tidy up any loose ends.

Physically, we were to engage in a strict diet for one week, two if we could, which meant excluding caffeine, meat, sugar, salt and dairy. Natasja explained in the preparation guide:

> We know that stress, fatigue, unbalanced diet: those excesses are reflected throughout the body. If the body is often maltreated by an unbalanced diet or too rich, this diet before the retreat is going to start to clean your body and will ensure you get the most out of your experience. You will have a sense of lightness and clarity which potentially gives you an opportunity to explore deeper . . .

Physical preparation also included being well rested, well slept and whatever exercise we needed to do to feel our best. Spiritually, Natasja advised that meditation could 'bring a higher vibrational spiritual energy to begin the purification process and to cultivate self-awareness'.

'Set and setting' are the most common buzz words in the psychedelic world and the best insurance against a 'bad trip'. Following Natasja's instructions to prepare ourselves for the ceremonies would ensure a wholesome 'mindset' while the retreat itself provided the ideal 'setting'. Psychedelics become more dangerous if we neglect set and setting and forget to respect the plants as sacred teachers.

Thoughts in the anticipation

Would I be the exception? The only one for whom mushrooms did not work their usual miracles? I suppose I harboured doubt due to my first attempt, in my living room, at taking psilocybin but also due to my relationship with alcohol. With drinking, I always found that any high was more than offset by hours of low energy, low mood and insomnia. Two cocktails at lunch would see me giggling like a schoolgirl—which was great—but the comedown robbed me of energy for hours afterwards and sometimes made me so cranky that abstinence seemed the best option.

Discussing all this with Luke he stated, 'I haven't noticed much abstinence from you.'

This was true, I never gave up trying, wondering if maybe this time would be different. Occasionally it was, but rarely.

'The last time I drank wine socially,' I complained, 'it made me so sleepy that I spent the whole evening faking wakefulness . . . It's such a social handicap for me,' I continued. 'You're lucky. You have a perfect relationship with alcohol. It makes you happy and the more you drink, the happier you get.'

'Up to a certain point, yes,' Luke conceded.

'But you know where that point is. You know when to stop, so alcohol has oiled a brilliant social life for you, full of camaraderie and happy memories.'

'I'm sure you're not the only one who needs to drink less as they get older,' Luke offered.

'Sure, a few friends have cut down, but we're a minority,' I said, adding, 'Not that you have to drink to have fun, but it sure helps socially.'

I hoped psychedelics could be my thing, or the thing that could help me feel more connected to my fellow humans.

Intentions

From the first Zoom preparation meeting, Natasja had encouraged us to reflect on what intentions we would bring to the psilocybin ceremonies. At this unique stage in my life, I had no major problems to address but plenty of pesky, self-inflicted ones. I decided to brainstorm some intentions by making a list of what I'd change about myself. Without coming up for breath I generated a list of 28 items (included in Appendix 1).

Natasja had encouraged us to come up with a positive intention rather than a negative; for example, instead of saying 'I will stop getting so stressed and anxious', we could say 'I will live more calmly'.

I settled on these four:

1. I will experience the Buddhist ideal of ego dissolution, leave my body and abandon the conventional self.
2. I will become calmer, lighter, floatier, more relaxed in all my muscles in daily life.
3. I will feel easier in my relations with others. I will delight more in their company and feel confident and comfortable in my own skin.
4. I will feel more relaxed and forgiving with a certain person I have failed to forgive (despite years of trying).

I was tempted to add a fifth but was starting to feel like I may already have too many:

5. I will feel more proud of myself, confident and accepting of my limitations.

I asked Natasja over Zoom, 'Is there a limit to how many intentions you can have?'

'I wouldn't get too hung up on the right number,' answered Natasja. 'Let the medicine decide. The plants decide which part of your mind they're going to work with.'

'You make it sound like the psilocybin is an entity in itself with its own personality,' I suggested.

'Oh, the plants are absolutely an entity with a personality—and sometimes they can be playful and fun.'

'Is it possible that none of my intentions will be fulfilled?' I asked.

'It's possible, although I will say the least likely of your intentions to be fulfilled is probably the first one: ego death.'

Natasja would explain, more than once, that the medicines often need to 'clean us out' of blockages, traumas and long-suppressed tension—before the spiritual awakenings can occur.

Bessel van der Kolk

A month or two before I left for Amsterdam, I attended a webinar presented by Bessel van der Kolk run by Mind Medicine Australia (more about this organisation in Chapter 21). I'd read his book *The Body Keeps the Score*, the definitive book on trauma, which explains that we store trauma in our bodies and, as such, we need to focus on the body as part of therapy. I often quoted from his book with my clients who, as victims of crime, had experienced trauma.[1] It's always amazing to come across someone you know of from work at an 'extracurricular activity', so hearing him talk about psychedelics was a treat.

He admitted that as a 'child of the sixties' he'd taken LSD, as had all his scientist friends and it'd been a life-changing experience. He claimed that the consensus among his friends was that it made them more 'creative scientists', for they learned that 'reality is so much larger than my little mind can conceive'.

In recent times, he had to take MDMA for his work and was most surprised at the effects. Before that he had never felt particularly affected by 'vicarious trauma', the trauma that those who work with the traumatised end up feeling in themselves. When he took

MDMA he learned that he had in fact been storing trauma. As he put it, 'over the eight hours, the thousands of traumatised people I've worked with came to visit me and I felt all the pain I have been carrying for them—I lay there for eight hours feeling their pain'.

Part of the secret of doing my job, working with victims of crime, was pushing it all aside in my spare time. I compartmentalised. I certainly didn't want any memories from work arising during my annual leave in the Netherlands. So I hoped that what happened to Bessel van der Kolk wouldn't happen to me.

I'd been working in the criminal justice system for almost five years and prior to that I'd worked in child protection for three or four. I'd seen a lot of suffering. My caseload is always over 100 cases—that's a lot of sad stories. The criminal justice system can be brutal to survivors of sexual assault who made up 90 per cent of my caseload. Some survivors even say their experience with the criminal justice system was worse than the original crime. We hear the word 're-traumatising' often. A large amount of the trauma comes from being cross-examined by a defence lawyer; read: being bullied for being sexually assaulted. On rare occasions, defence lawyers are polite and respectful, but more often they have a contemptuous manner—sneering even—as they try to paint the victim as a liar.

The victims often need breaks as they give their evidence, to go and cry. Some get angry but juries tend to punish that. I have read hundreds of victim impact statements and I understand that the degree of damage a sexual assault can do to a person's soul is immeasurable. Yet victim impact statements are written only by the victims who obtain a guilty verdict. It's especially disturbing that so many victims suffer a sexual assault, give evidence, survive cross-examination, only to receive a Not Guilty verdict. I've always felt so sad for them. Yet at the end of the day, I can switch off. I do feel people's pain deeply; I'm just able to move on—or I couldn't do the job.

As it turned out, what happened to Bessel van der Kolk on MDMA was exactly what would happen to me on psilocybin. The body does keep the score.

3

Psilocybin in the Netherlands

I WANDER AROUND AMSTERDAM airport, the meeting place from where a shuttle bus will take us an hour north to a country home for our five-day retreat. I'm an hour early, to avoid the stress of being late, and my stomach is doing flips at the thought of meeting so many strangers at once—an overwhelming prospect for any introvert, admittedly made easier by three hours' worth of Zoom meetings behind us.

The Netherlands decided to ban mushrooms in 2008 after a seventeen-year-old French girl, in the Netherlands on a school excursion, died by suicide, jumping from a building after eating psilocybin mushrooms.[1] No toxicology report ever materialised to prove she'd taken mushrooms.

Despite the ban, a legal loophole left room for the part of the mushroom that grows *under* the ground, the less potent 'truffle', to remain legal. Thanks to that loophole, retreats flourish and smartshops abound selling psilocybin truffles, cannabis products and other natural medicines.

The Netherlands is one of an increasing number of countries that has a drug-checking service. Their Drug Information and Monitoring System, established in the 1990s, allows users of any drug to test its purity at one of thirty-one sites around the country.[2] Since July 2022, Australia has had one pill-testing centre, located in Canberra, CanTEST Health and Drug Checking Service, open for three hours on a Thursday and three hours on a Friday. In the first month, of 58 samples submitted for testing, users disposed of eighteen of them that were deemed too risky to consume.[3]

Who was on the retreat?

There had been nothing to fear: each retreatant had felt nervous, like me, but all still managed to present as warm, friendly and excited about the days ahead. The group comprised seven men and four women, including me, all from English-speaking countries except one Swiss man and one Spaniard who both spoke perfect English. I was towards the upper end of the age range but there was nobody in their twenties.

For some reason, they were an entrepreneurial bunch, most of them ran their own businesses in areas like music promotion, climate action, plumbing and corporate training. I was definitely the only public servant—and the only person with a boss. As the days went by, I would be struck at how almost everyone expressed deep love, and gratitude, for their partner back home. Including me. This happened to be unusual in my experience.

As eleven perfect strangers there would be no cliques but a level playing field where we all came from a different part of the world. Admittedly, three of the men had already been on one of Natasja's retreats. This was reassuring—repeat business for Natasja was an unsurpassable endorsement and all three said words to the effect: 'I'd trust Natasja with my life' and 'Natasja is the safest pair of hands in this space'.

To be in the hands of this inspiring team, and among such kindred spirits, would be invaluable to the set and setting of the ceremonies ahead.

Set and setting on the retreat

After a couple of days, I made a sneaky phone call to Luke, back home. Phone use was discouraged, but I knew he was alone, without the company he'd recently grown used to since I moved in with him.

'So, what's it like?' Luke asked.

'It's amazing. Everyone here—Natasja's team, the other people on the retreat—they're all excited and super-friendly and everyone has a great sense of humour so we're laughing a lot and sharing pretty deeply too. I'm really enjoying getting to know them all. Everyone's embracing the experience a hundred per cent.'

'What's the place like?'

'Let's see, it's a two-storey, rustic home with ten or so bedrooms and about three living rooms or activity rooms. It's set in rambling fields with irrigation canals running through them and all these exotic birds. We've been on a walk through the fields—it's cold, though.'

'Yeah, Sydney's been in the mid-twenties. So, what kind of things have you been doing, darling?'

'Oh, I've been in my element. The program's been full of all my favourite things like dancing, meditation, sharing circles where you truly connect to each other. Each day starts with a session of qi gong, which is a bit like meditation with gentle movements.'

We participated in the 'sharing circles' as a whole group and also in smaller groups, or pairs, as opportunities to reflect on our 'internal weather'. What I liked best was that we used a 'talking stick': whoever held it, would not be interrupted until the gong sounded and the next person received the stick. As a small woman with a slight invisibility complex, I appreciated the rare opportunity to talk without being interrupted, with space to pause and collect my thoughts without someone interrupting. I also enjoyed listening to the other retreatants as they too shared with compelling honesty.

Luke was a patient conversationalist. I didn't want to ask him about life back in Sydney and leave the bubble I was in, so this conversation was *all about me*. I had to tie up the call soon as I could hear my roommate finishing her shower in our bathroom.

'I'm feeling nourished, nurtured and spiritually spoilt,' I concluded. 'The food's delicious and everything smells heavenly—they use all these scents and oils and shamanic incense. Smoking sage, I believe.'

The facilitators had certainly created a sensual feast: along with the aromas were petals, feathers, candles, shamanic trinkets and a carefully curated playlist of tribal, spiritual and classical music.

A cacao ceremony

Psilocybin ceremonies would not be the only means of altering our consciousness on the retreat. We gathered into a circle in one of the activity rooms where Natasja introduced cacao:

> Pure cacao is used as a heart-opening medicine for people to safely experience awakening, revelation and inner healing. It's also used to set intentions and once consumed, euphoric states are unlocked, negative emotions are released, and we are able to connect to ourselves and the loving energy in our body.

We drank the cacao as a tea, made from the crushed beans, and before long I felt the euphoria. All feeling aglow, we engaged in an array of joyful activities: drawing with coloured pencils, dancing to exotic music and taking turns to share with the group our present feelings and our dreams for the future. Of course, cacao is no psychedelic and it's perfectly legal all around the world. I made a mental note to stock up on cacao nibs when I arrived home.

Psilocybin Ceremony one

Natasja always referred to her team of four as space holders, who would 'hold', or ensure, a safe space, ever vigilant to anything we journeyers might need in a given moment. Before we entered the ceremony room a space holder performed the ancient Native American ritual of 'smudging' each one of us, which acted to purify us to prepare for the ceremony. One by one, we held our arms out straight to the side and a space holder moved a branch of sage with aromatic, smouldering leaves around the perimeter of our bodies. The cleansing ritual, together with the heavenly smell, reinforced the sacred nature of what we were about to partake in.

We filed into the carefully prepared room, with its shamanic ornaments, candles, cushions and blankets and each sat on a thin mattress, backs to the wall against a pillow. The space holders sat up the front, on a slightly raised platform, to take care of us and attend to any needs that might arise such as giving us moral support, or water or guiding us to the bathroom when wobbly on our feet. The space holders on their cushions looked so picturesque, all dressed in white, the scene could have been an album cover: *Songs of Healing* by The Space Holders.

I felt only calm about what I was about to do. As we went round the group, each retreatant shared how they felt, and I reported no fear.

'I'm excited!' I announced. 'I've done my research and know the medicine's safe. Even if I have a so-called bad trip, I'll learn something helpful. I have faith I'll get the journey I need.'

After some shamanic prayers, we each received a mug, wherein lay a tea with some truffles at the bottom.

It was time to drink.

The truffles tasted nutty but not bitter.

A few tracks into the playlist, the medicine took effect. A light show: a stream of bright colours, mosaics, patterns moved and changed in quick succession. 'Sacred geometry,' as it's often called. Incredibly beautiful and compelling. I was happy already.

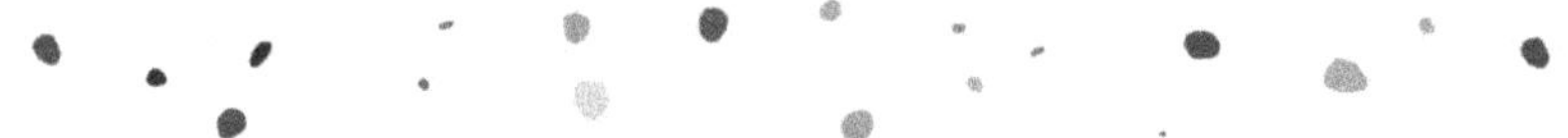

I feel an energy-force thump through me. I'm shaking and spasming, in a stream of sudden, jerky movements. What is going on with my body? Why, oh why, am I shaking and writhing? It feels dramatic and I'm sure it looks dramatic. I'm consumed with curiosity—and then it hits me: I'm in labour. I'm giving birth to something. Even my breathing is that of a woman in labour—the fast panting, the blowing with the mouth, yet no pain. My body moves violently with the effort of giving birth but now something different again begins. The energy reverses direction. It goes from the push, push, push of giving birth to receiving energy from the other direction. What on earth is that? Then I realise, with dismay: it's the feeling of being raped.

As though my body is under anaesthetic, I feel none of the sensations that a true victim of sexual assault feels, only the pounding. I notice above me, in neon lights, the three letters that denote the organisation I work for: actual signage, in case of any doubt, confirms that this relates to my work. I'm processing the trauma of the victims of sexual assault.

The faces of three victims pass repeatedly before my eyes. I'm anaesthetised, so I'm strong enough to bear their pain, share their turmoil. I'm relieving them of some of the immense emotional burden. I know that I can bear this because the mushrooms help me. I'm working through scores and scores of the victims, 'taking it' for them, so that the burden of their pain can be shared and not down to one lone woman to carry.

The energy suddenly reverses direction and I'm back to labour, the pushing and pushing, the breathing quickly and puffing. The two experiences keep switching every few minutes: pushing out, pounding, pushing out, pounding. The pounding I understand, but what am I giving birth to? What is going to come out of me? I feel frustrated with the not-knowing.

It's been hours of this, and I become irritated by the spasms. I stand up and lean against the wall—maybe that will make it stop. It doesn't. It doesn't feel horrific or distressing, just something my body needs to work through.

Numerous images of my second-born, Alex, appear: the moment of his birth, the first latch on to my breast, him as a toddler repeating 'labradoodle' and many images of him dancing, as a toddler, as a child, as a teenager. I hug him again and again and tell him I love him and repeatedly mouth the words, 'Alex is all there is, Alex is all there is.' Tears of love spill from me. I bliss out.

Suddenly, I perceive that Alex has died. I see a coffin carried through a crowd. I continue crying, please don't let this be true. Has he killed himself while I'm here in Amsterdam? Or is this an omen that he will eventually kill himself? I hug him continually and keep him close to me, his face smiles at me. Why do I feel so certain of his death, or imminent death? 'It's okay, mum,' he says, 'I'm here.'

•

I see the face of Sam—who I've been trying to forgive for decades. A stream of images: Sam looking lost, Sam looking out-of-control, scared. Now Sam stands alone in a cavernous, dark, empty room. Sam cries, hands over face, shoulders quaking, racked with the pain of suffering. My heart swings open. If compassion is a verb, I'm compassioning hard. All I want to do is comfort this suffering human being. I put an arm around Sam's quivering body to provide comfort to the grief.

Now Sam is alone at a dinner table, simply eating lunch, and I'm struck by Sam's loneliness and isolation. Every movement Sam makes eating that sandwich feels poignant, sweet and childlike. I'm overcome by the vulnerability and gripped by the certainty that Sam needs human connection. I can provide it. I will provide it. This is my purpose.

What if this realisation disappears just as fast as it came? I determine to stay with Sam. I need to give Sam some time in order to make the feeling stay, so I lie next to Sam on a couch holding hands, feeling close. I've been searching for this feeling, this love for Sam, for so many years and now I feel a sense of deep peace as we lie together.

The ceremony ends

We all gradually land back in the room and share a need to stand up and stretch our legs after about six or seven hours of sitting. The music takes off and we dance and hug each other before sitting again for a brief sharing circle—without going into the finer details of our journeys. Everyone in the room has experienced something different.

'I didn't experience any visuals,' one man shared. Visuals had felt like two hours for me.

'I mainly experienced hours of crying—tears of joy and gratitude actually,' he said.

'I managed to forgive someone I've been angry with for decades,' I shared. 'I just hope it sticks.'

There were two retreatants who sounded a little disappointed with their experience, but they were both comparing their journey to some prior journey, as one of them said: 'It was nothing like my experience on 5-MeO-DMT. That blew my socks off and changed my life. I wanted that to happen again, but it didn't.' 5-MeO-DMT was the psychedelic collected from a toad and which provided an extremely powerful trip of around half an hour.

'At one point in the trip,' shared one man, 'I wasn't sure if I was hallucinating or whether there was a fire in the room.'

There had in fact been a fire in the room when a blanket fell on a candle. It never amounted to much of a conflagration as one of the space holders quickly extinguished it. A space holder's role, after all, is to put out fires, literally and figuratively.

I was exhausted from the trip, which ended at around 8 p.m. but ever the insomniac, I didn't sleep all night. At least I had some time to review my journey.

Integration with Natasja

One of the first things I did after the psilocybin ceremony was send Alex a message to reassure myself that he was alive. He replied that he was at work, on a long shift, and could he borrow the car?

Thankfully, I would soon be able to discuss my trip in a one-to-one with Natasja, thus beginning the all-important step of Integration. Many in the psychedelic world believe that the work we do after taking a psychedelic—the discussions, therapy, journalling, reflection and attention to our bodies—is more important than the trip itself. We sat on some cushions on the floor of the ceremony room a couple of days later.

'I say to everyone,' Natasja began, 'I don't have all the answers. I won't be able to tell you what it all means.'

'I'm confused,' I told Natasja. 'I thought the medicine revealed great truths, but Alex hasn't died. Will he die soon? How am I to take this? I felt so sure that he'd died.'

'Well, we're all going to die.' Natasja smiled.

I gave Natasja some background, 'Alex has had some real suffering in his life and even though life generally goes quite well for him, there have been times when I've worried that he might decide to end it all, even though I knew it was unlikely. He's definitely caused me anxiety as he was quite the troubled teenager, changing schools twice.'

'Our fears and worries are highly likely to be amplified by the medicines,' Natasja replied. 'Don't take what you experience too literally. Sometimes it's just an invitation to find new ways to work with things.'

'Well, I'm so keen to know what it means,' I said as I moved on to the next theme, revealing that I spent the trip alternating between giving birth and being raped. 'I understand the rape part—that relates to my job, but what about giving birth?' I asked.

'I suspect the two experiences are linked,' Natasja replied. 'Particularly on my women's retreats, I have worked with retreatants who were psychologists and counsellors and I've found they're carrying the traumas of their clients and that these traumas can interact with their own. Being in labour is a familiar experience for your body so is probably a known way, a go-to, for it to process all the trauma you have experienced at work. In the ancient mystery schools, a woman's womb isn't just seen as the portal for creation but also for destruction, chaos and death.'

'It's like Bessel van der Kolk's book *The Body Keeps the Score,'* I suggested. 'My body has stored stress or vicarious trauma and the psilocybin has helped release it.'

'The spasms were a way to release blocked energy, or a way for your nervous system to release tension,' Natasja continued. There had been talk throughout the retreat about how animals in the wild, after a chase, shake and tremble to process stress in their bodies.

'I guess it's great that I released these traumas from my body but what can I do about the future if I stay at my job—my body will just keep collecting trauma, won't it?'

'It might be worth looking into somatic processing,' Natasja suggested. Why had I never heard these two words? 'Processing trauma,' Natasja continued, 'needs to include your body, so you might like to look into breath or body work or consulting with a somatic counsellor as a way to release the tensions.'

'I've been doing my job for five years, Natasja, maybe it's time to give myself a break? Maybe it isn't sustainable for me, for too much longer.' I half hoped Natasja would tell me to quit.

'Keep in mind,' Natasja warned, 'we all need to avoid making big decisions in the early days after the retreat.'

This is the same advice I'd heard in the closing of Buddhist retreats I'd attended.

'I'm curious,' Natasja asked, 'to know about the forgiveness you experienced on the journey—you mentioned it to the group?'

I reminded her of my fourth intention, to forgive a certain person.

'In the past, I could forgive Sam with my head,' I explained, 'but not with my heart. I was too hurt and caught up in trying to make sense of the behaviour: "How could Sam do this to me? Why? Why?".'

'What do you think made it click?' Natasja asked.

'I realised it's not about me anymore and surrendered my bruised ego. I felt this happen on a deep level, or in my heart, not my head. I was able to get out of the way and I feel like it's the start of a new phase in the relationship.'

For years I'd tried to reason my way out of my resentment towards Sam. I'd focused on her when I'd attended one Buddhist retreat, meditating about her, trying to understand how any past suffering for her may explain the actions that had hurt me. I even raised it in a discussion with one of the Buddhist teachers who replied: 'It sounds like you perceive the situation as a collection of little boxes, tightly wrapped up in brown paper, fastened with sticky tape and tied up with string. The situation may not be as fixed as you perceive it to be. Maybe you could unwrap some of those boxes and even throw some away.'

I'd liked her metaphor, but I also thought that it may have been something she could say to everyone who came to speak to her, about anything. Not that this necessarily lessened its value. Her words helped, but, alas, I would continue to carry a grudge for another decade or more. Until psilocybin.

Breathwork session

The day after the first psilocybin ceremony, we did a session on breathwork, as a way to potentially alter our consciousness. A therapist from Amsterdam, Katrien taught us a breathing technique, but my nose was blocked, and I couldn't do it for more than a few minutes due to my dry throat. I gave up, tuned out and treated myself to a meditation instead. To my surprise, meditating after even a little breathwork gave rise to one of the most focused meditation sessions I've ever experienced. My mind wandered so much less than usual. I made a mental note to start all my meditation sessions from that point on with deep, slow breathing.

I looked round the room at the other retreatants during the breathwork session and assumed the activity was a little underwhelming, that it wasn't working for anyone. Imagine my surprise when it came time for the group to share: one after another, people described amazing experiences, realisations and epiphanies. I would need to give breathwork another chance at a later date.

There was one more psilocybin ceremony to take place on the retreat. The first in no way prepared me for what was in store in the second.

4

Second psilocybin ceremony

I WAS SEVERELY SLEEP-DEPRIVED for the second ceremony on day four, but I wasn't the only one. I also had a head cold that required nose-blowing every two minutes, so I worried I'd disturb the journeys of others with my cold-related noise. Despite these small problems, I felt euphoric from the afterglow of the first ceremony and the joy of the retreat.

The space holders smudged each one of us with the smoking sage before we re-entered the ceremony room and sat in our circle to prepare.

I asked, 'There seem to be a few of us behind on sleep. Does that matter?'

'Even better,' Natasja replied cheerfully. 'Being tired increases the chances you'll surrender to the experience.'

I drank down my tea and waited a couple of minutes for the journey to begin. It started with the mesmerising visuals but I perceived them at an awkward angle I was powerless to adjust. I enjoyed the colour show but wanted something more to happen. It did.

I receive a powerful message about my ex-husband, 'Marek must do this retreat.' I repeat this message to myself twenty times—I mustn't forget to tell him. It's important.

Now I'm no longer in the same room with the group and I notice space holders Karen and Henk sitting on either side of me. 'It's okay,' I say to them. 'I get the message. Marek must do this.'

'Who is Mark?' asks Henk.

'It's not Mark, it's Marek,' I say bossily. 'He's Polish. Marek is the Polish form of Mark.'

'Who is he to you?' asks Henk.

'He's my ex-husband and he's been a refugee, and he had some real suffering in life growing up in Poland and he has to do this retreat.'

'Do you think Marek would do a retreat like this?' Henk asks.

'Um . . . probably not,' I was clear enough to say.

'This is *your* time now,' Henk says. 'Why don't you concentrate on what you need?'

I turn to Karen.

'It's okay,' I assure her. 'I've got the message now and I absolutely promise I'll tell him to come here and do this.'

Still sitting with Karen and Henk, outside the main room, I feel a deep peace descend on me, a strong sense that I've crossed over into another realm. It's an encounter with the Divine, not that I hear or see anything divine, but I strongly sense the presence. It's a 'them', rather than a single entity. The Divine is plural. I'm on the 'other side' and when Karen and Henk escort me back to the room with the other retreatants, I feel reluctant to return to my life, especially my work life, back in Australia. I'm happy here in this new realm. I have a sense that everything about life back on Earth is absurd, except the love I feel for those precious to me.

Given the absurdity, I have the insight that I can go back to my life and hold everything more loosely, not take things so seriously. Nothing matters nearly as much as I usually believe it does. Leave it all to the universe and stop trying to control everything.

'I don't have to go back, do I?' I ask Karen and Henk who start escorting me back to the main room.

'Yes,' Karen laughed.

On re-entering the ceremony space, everyone's eyes are open again, as the trip has ended for most. They all look at me with a kind smile. I have no idea why.

The journey ends

Gradually I felt myself return to the room. Suddenly I remembered I'd made a fool of myself. When sitting with Henk and Karen outside the room, I'd thought Henk was a painting. I'd reached out to touch his face. Startled, he had flinched back as both space holders gasped in surprise. Now that the trip was over, I realised how that must have looked. He must have seen it as an attempt at affection—or worse. Oh, how excruciatingly embarrassing. I started laughing every time I thought of it.

As we all gradually landed back in reality, the music from the playlist went up in tempo and Natasja started dancing, joined by most of the euphoric retreatants. Some just wanted to hug everyone. One retreatant started singing and the beauty of her voice—her early career had been in musical theatre—left me awe-struck. As though I wasn't already at maximum levels of awe.

In the post-journey sharing circle, I apologised to Henk. He brushed it off, like a gentleman.

Dissociation

If my account of the second ceremony seems shorter than the first, it's because something bizarre happened.

At the end of the trip, as everyone chatted, hugged and milled around, at least three people approached me and said: 'It was really hard not to go over and help you. I wanted to reach out to you, but I knew it wasn't the thing to do.'

Another couple of people came up to me, separately, and told me how they felt so relieved when I returned to the room, as the group felt incomplete without me.

I had no idea what they were talking about. I started asking people why I'd been taken from the room, knowing full well that it could only have been for making a helluva commotion. I inquired of the man who sat next to me who said, 'You were just sobbing.'

'For how long?' I asked.

'About two hours.'

'Two hours?' I blurted, in disbelief.

'Probably longer,' chimed in another retreatant.

'But I don't remember making the slightest noise,' I responded. 'I have no idea why I was even making noise.'

All kinds of feedback came my way. One man offered, 'I thought you were having orgasms or giving birth or something.'

Nice to know I kept my dignity.

Needless to say, I was dying to find out what had happened to me. I was the only person the space holders had decided to take from the room. During my one-to-one integration session with Natasja, my first question was: 'Why can't I remember what happened to me? It's like I blacked out.'

'There's a chance that you dissociated,' she replied.

'But why? Do you know?'

'It sometimes happens when your nervous system, or your psyche, is overwhelmed. Maybe you weren't ready to be present for your trauma. The kind of noise you were making during the journey sounded like a crying baby.' She imitated the cry a tired baby makes when they sound a little disengaged from their crying but they're giving it one last shot before falling asleep.

'But why would I cry like a baby?'

'You might've been reliving your birth,' Natasja suggested. 'That's a very common experience with the medicines. I've seen it several times before and experienced it myself.' Maybe that would explain why I felt like I was viewing the visuals at an awkward angle. Perhaps I'd been starting a journey down the birth canal.

'Do you know anything about the details of your birth?' Natasja asked.

'No, I don't. Does it suggest I had a traumatic birth?'

'Every birth's traumatic. Then again, you may have dissociated from an experience of feeling abandoned as a baby. Maybe after you were delivered the nurses took you somewhere rather than letting you be with your mother—they knew less about what babies needed back then. Or maybe as a baby when you cried you didn't get the attention you needed.'

I cast my mind back searching for answers—and found one. 'I remember when my first baby, Zac, was crying,' I told Natasja, 'my mother mentioned that when I was a baby she'd just leave me to cry it out.'

I would soon discuss this time with my mother who explained how she was dying to go and comfort her babies but tried to follow the advice of the day and teach us to 'self-settle'. Parents were to avoid rewarding the crying with attention so that babies could learn to fall asleep by themselves, my mother explained. By the time my babies arrived the advice was similar but added the need to comfort the crying baby at regular intervals.

Then I thought of another explanation. 'One of my earliest memories,' I told Natasja, 'is screaming hysterically in my bed wanting my mother to come, and getting really wound up when she didn't.' Of course, I've never blamed my mother for this. I was a sleep-shy toddler who always resisted bedtime and kicked up a stink every night about going to bed. I don't blame her for leaving me to cry from time to time, for the sake of her sanity, and in the hope that I'd eventually self-settle. I can't remember clearly but suspect I may have left Alex to cry on occasion when he was a toddler due to the sheer amount of time he spent crying.

Questions still tormented me. What's the point of an experience that you're not even present for—how can I learn from that?

A few more trips into my psychedelic journey, further light would be shed on my infancy.

Failing to make sense of the message

My second trip felt like being repeatedly dumped by waves at the beach. There'd been nausea, wrist pain, a chaotic series of emotions and a complete blackout or 'dissociation'.

It felt like the whole trip had been about ensuring Marek came on this retreat. Yet when the trip had worn off, I felt confused. I knew Marek would never in a million years do this retreat. These were not his people. Why was so much of my trip spent on this message? I even felt mildly resentful that this had taken up so much space—surely there were more important messages than this one that I knew would never lead to anything.

To do this retreat you had to be prepared to work on yourself. Marek had never read even a page of a self-help book—even though I'd written five of them while we were together, one of them about our marriage. He couldn't have been less interested in personal development let alone spiritual growth. Since our breakup we'd become the best of friends—I had a good handle on my baggage. So why did he feature in my trip? I was flummoxed and dying to run it by Natasja.

Natasja is not above saying, 'I don't know', and in the case of Marek she couldn't tell me why I received this message.

'I'm so confused. Can the plants mess with you, or even bully you?'

'The plants don't bully you—they show you your shadow side, the parts that you haven't addressed. Sometimes the plants present us with metaphors or new ways of looking at our lives. We don't have to take everything literally.'

This resonated. It was why religious texts were full of parables, or stories, as this allows us to choose from an array of interpretations.

'So, I guess I just have to accept that, for now, there's no answer to why I received this message so strongly?' I pressed.

'Sometimes it takes years for things to make sense. Once it was twelve years before I realised what one of my journeys was about. As long as we go into a journey mentally stable, we can trust the process. It will unfold in its own good time.'

I'd eventually meet a man called Carlos, originally an engineer like Marek, whose childhood friend had tracked him down after receiving a strong message during a trip that 'Carlos must take this medicine'. Today, Carlos is no longer an engineer and runs ayahuasca retreats (see Chapter 12 for his full story). This was an unlikely outcome for Marek.

Closing advice to the group

In our last group meeting on the retreat, I told the group: 'I couldn't believe the empathy and care you all expressed towards me at the end of the second trip. If someone sat next to me sobbing for over two hours, I can't guarantee that empathy is what I'd feel. Next time I feel irritated by people's noise, I'll remember the model you've provided.'

On another note, Natasja advised: 'Don't tell people back home too much about what happened during your journeys. Their reactions might influence how the memory sits with you. When you tell a story several times it loses its intensity.'

I was relieved to hear this advice as I knew people back home might ask me about my trips and I had no desire to present them over and over again before I'd processed them myself.

Alexander Beiner, the co-facilitator of the retreat, added: 'Don't grow too obsessed with meaning-making or with trying to make sense of your journeys. Just accept that often there is a gradual "unfolding" of the experience. One day I was sitting on a couch when—boom!—I suddenly understood what my experience meant on a journey I'd had years ago.'

Amsterdam

The retreat was over, and I'd organised to spend a few days in Amsterdam to rest, digest the experience and continue the process of integration. For the first day I didn't leave my hotel room until late afternoon. I was exhausted but also wanted to hold on to the feelings, the afterglow. I was amazed to find the spasms from my first trip recurring every few hours. As I wrote up my trip reports, I'd take breaks to lie on my bed and let a few more spasms course through me.

I also called Alex that day to discuss his death, and he said: 'Oh, I know what was happening there. I've moved out. The old Alex, the little boy you had to look after, is dead and gone.'

'Why didn't I think of that?' I replied, 'I think you're probably spot on.'

Next, I called Marek. I knew exactly how he'd respond to the message for him. He'd chuckle and brush it off—and that's exactly what he did.

That day, I tapped out 4000 words, a personal best for a day's work. I felt as though something was working through me. It all spilled out of me effortlessly, as though I was merely the typist, and the plants were working through me. I had no idea if a publisher would accept the idea I'd submitted to write a book about my psychedelic experiences, but my first retreat had been so fascinating that it helped me to believe a book contract was a distinct possibility.

It already felt as though this book would write itself. It reminded me of the TED Talk by Elizabeth Gilbert, author of *Eat, Pray, Love*, where she spoke of how the ancient Greeks and Romans believed creativity did not come from any individual human but from a 'divine attendant spirit that came to human beings from some distant and unknowable source for distant and unknowable reasons'. In those days creatives *had* a genius to help them with the creative process and provide the ideas, then the assumptions of society changed, and people could *be* a genius themselves.

The second day after the retreat I was curious to visit one of the twelve smartshops that sold psilocybin and other magic powders and potions—and see the sights of Amsterdam. Striding out of my hotel, I was struck first by the absence of cars and the large number of bicycles, with riders of all ages. Dutch architecture has perfect consistency—who knew brown buildings could look so attractive? With a third of the country below sea level, the city is built on over a million poles up to 12 metres long and this is why some of the canal houses tilt. Houseboats line the canals as if living on the water is a perfectly normal lifestyle choice. The Dutch make me feel like a blotchy dwarf as they're all inhumanly tall—with the average Dutch man at 6 foot—and their complexions don't often see the sun.

A steady drizzle of light rain while I was there was not enough to inspire anyone to bust out an umbrella or a raincoat—they had all learned to overlook this level of wetness. I wouldn't see a ray of sunshine in my five days there and was told by the recording on the canal cruise that when the sun comes out, the Dutch drag chairs out of their houses to sit on the street absorbing the rays. Despite the weather, and Anne Frank's hideout, there's a feel-good vibe, from the outdoor ice-skating rink to the art galleries of the Great Masters, all endorsed by plenty of tourists, many of whom sport wide grins and smell like cannabis, having visited a 'coffee shop'. I've got a friend who walked into one searching for a salt- and sugar-free meal; she showed her confused face to everyone assembled, before slinking out.

Eventually, I stumbled on a smartshop that had a red-topped, white-spotted mushroom as signage, not that any psilocybin mushrooms have red tops, but the red-tops are pretty and make a good logo. I bought a T-shirt with one such mushroom on it, and hoped the shop assistants would let me ply them with questions. The fresh-faced man at the counter, whose curls snaked out from under his beanie, seemed open to an interview.

'I always ask customers who buy mushrooms, "Are you looking for a high or an introspective experience?" Most are looking for a high.'

'What percentage would you say?' I asked.

'I'd say 80 per cent of customers who buy mushrooms are just looking for fun.'

'Why do you think that is?'

'There's a lack of good information out there. People don't realise the potential of psilocybin to change your life. Mushrooms are useful for getting to know your dark side. That's how I got this job—I understand that potential from my own experiences.'

His colleague approached and my eyes roamed around his face noting piercings in places I didn't know you could have them.

I asked him, 'How do people treat you when you tell them what you do for a living?'

'Mixed,' he replied. 'When my university lecturer found out, he said he'd visit next weekend and could I give him a discount. Other people just write me off as some druggo.'

Lost in the streets a little later, I asked a young Thai man for directions. We soon found ourselves in a conversation and I learned his name was Ter and he was a software engineer in Belgium, in Amsterdam for the weekend to smoke some weed with a friend. He was interested to hear about my retreat and shared that he'd had a bad trip with a substance called ketamine, which is technically a dissociative, but at high doses can have psychedelic effects. He said he thought he was going to die and had feared for his life. Despite this, he asked me to come along with him back to the smartshop as he was open to trying some mushrooms.

About two weeks after I left Amsterdam, I received a text from Ter:

> Hi Sarah, I just took the mushroom this morning in my room after waking up. It was brilliant. Now I get you about getting to know yourself.

I replied:

> I'm so glad it was a good experience. Did you get the visuals you were hoping for? What did you learn about yourself, if it's not a personal question?

Ter then wrote:

> Yes, I saw those visuals, in and outside of my head, it was amazing. I did learn to love myself more. I saw myself or

> things that remind me back in times in pieces, it was not as clear as a movie but I recognise it. It's a rollercoaster. Hard to explain.

I did relate to what Ter said about seeing himself 'back in times in pieces' as I too had seen many random, unconnected images from my past. I texted him:

> Wow, that's probably the most common thing you hear actually, that it's hard to explain what happened. It's all a bit beyond language . . .

That said, there is a website called Erowid where hundreds of people have written trip reports after taking a psychedelic. It receives 55,000 hits a day. In their 'Experience Vaults', trip reports are grouped in categories such as 'first time', 'difficult experiences' and 'mystical experiences'.[1]

Back in Sydney

Intrigued by the revelations of my psilocybin experience, I desperately wanted to continue the adventure and explore other psychedelic substances by writing a book. In equal measure, I was tired of all the routine and administrative tasks that dominated my public service job so I found myself compulsively checking my emails to see if the publisher I'd approached would give me the greenlight. In the weeks after the retreat, I enjoyed reunions through the 4 a.m. Zoom calls and found that since the retreat everyone was in some kind of honeymoon period of coping better with stress, deadlines and difficult people. Some of us regularly listened to the playlist from our trips to keep the retreat alive.

I had used the window of neuroplasticity after psilocybin to reinstate a daily meditation practice. Luke and I had always meditated together on Saturday and Sunday, but other than that I was lucky to squeeze another sit into my rushed working week. Following the retreat, a daily sit seemed crucial to the integration.

At the third integration call—three weeks after the retreat had ended—I shared my surprise at how much easier mindful living seemed: I now lived far more in the present, noticing my thoughts, reactions and moods. Mindfulness had always felt difficult to sustain, for any length of time, but now, in the psilocybin afterglow, it seemed effortless. I still felt extremely happy and woke up looking forward to the day ahead. Nevertheless, I wouldn't stay this high for much longer.

5

Lead-up to Bufo in Portugal

In the months after the psilocybin retreat, the effortless mindfulness, along with the happiness, would eventually fade. I knew that, after five years in my job, the exposure to sad stories was not sustainable for me, so when I eventually heard back from the publisher that they were prepared to offer me a contract to write a book about psychedelics, I quit my job immediately, giving six weeks' notice. I'd already booked my next retreat and the timing worked perfectly so that my last day would be the day before I left Australia.

In the afterglow of the psilocybin retreat, there was no doubt in my mind that I'd do another retreat with Natasja. Leaving three months between medicine journeys, as she'd recommended, I booked a trip to Portugal, Natasja's childhood home. This time the retreat was for the psychedelic Bufo, otherwise known as 5-MeO-DMT or 'toad'. Bufo is short for *Bufo alvarius*, the name of a toad found in the southwestern USA and northwestern Mexico. When its glands are squeezed, it's possible to collect its milky venom, a process which, happily, doesn't kill the toad. Still, the toad is endangered by the actions of the burgeoning numbers interested in their venom, so it's more responsible to use a synthetic form. Natasja had used both forms in the past, had observed no difference and cares deeply about any threat to the toad's future, so I'd take the synthetic form on the retreat.

Portugal and drugs

Portugal has long been an international superstar when it comes to drug policy. Back when I was a volunteer for Family Drug Support, over a decade ago, I constantly heard about how progressive and successful Portugal had been in addressing their drug problem. Once a country with a serious heroin issue, the government realised that the strategies of the war on drugs had failed. In the year 2000, Portugal boldly decriminalised all drugs, moving from an emphasis on punishment to treatment. Drug trafficking would still land you in gaol, but if you were caught with an amount deemed 'for personal use', you wouldn't be punished by the criminal justice system, but rather, stood before a panel of health professionals who might recommend any of a number of options including counselling, time in detox, community service, a fine or rehabilitation.

Before long, deaths from overdose were down, along with prison numbers, AIDS and drug-related crime. Treatment numbers were up, and Portugal became a case study for other countries to learn from, albeit slowly. While heroin use declined, there was an increase in experimentation with other drugs such as cannabis, but given decriminalisation, it had also become safer to admit to drug use when completing surveys—which may have inflated these figures. While decriminalisation was divisive in Portugal at the time, these days there's wide public support for the successful policy. Today, psychedelic retreats abound in Portugal and while the drugs may not be 'legal', they are 'decriminalised', and the justice system is yet to demonstrate any interest in the use of decriminalised substances on retreats.[1]

What does Bufo do?

Bufo is generally viewed as the psychedelic that provides the most powerful experience—Michael Pollan has referred to it as the Everest of psychedelics. He described his own experience of Bufo, however, as 'just horrible'. Bufo is similar in some fundamental ways to the psychedelic DMT, or Dimethyltryptamine, and is actually the same thing with a few extra atoms attached and different effects. They are similar in that they work on serotonin receptors and the effects begin almost instantly and last less than an hour. However, Bufo is described as four to six times stronger than DMT and provides the possibility, for some journeyers, of an experience of ego dissolution, or of merging with the universe.[2] DMT, on the other hand (discussed further in Chapter 19) is known for the likelihood of meeting a deity or an entity.

An Australian researcher, Dr Uthaug, has described Bufo as a 'somatic amplifier' inducing a cathartic, body-based experience where you release painful emotions and memories.[3] The release allows for a 'reset of the nervous system'. This describes what would happen to me.

A survey conducted by Johns Hopkins University researchers in 2018 found that taking Bufo led to improvements in anxiety and depression for 80 per cent of the 362 adults who tried it. As with other psychedelic studies, they found a strong correlation between such improvements and the intensity of the mystical experiences.[4] The key to the healing power of Bufo, as has been found with many psychedelics, may be in its ability to reveal aspects of a spiritual realm.

While indigenous tribes have used Bufo for millennia[5], Albert Most—real name: Ken Nelson—brought the medicine to light for Westerners. He made a pilgrimage to find the Bufo toad, and bravely try its venom. He eventually published a pamphlet in 1983 in which he described the journey:

> You will be completely absorbed in a complex chemical event characterized by an overload of thoughts and perception, brief collapse of the EGO, and loss of the space-time continuum. Relax, breathe regularly, and flow with the experience. After two to three minutes, the initial intensity fades to a pleasant LSD-like sensation in which visual illusions, hallucinations, and perceptual distortions are common. You may sense a distortion in your perceived body image or notice the world shrinking or expanding. You may notice that colours seem brighter and more

> beautiful than usual. And, most likely, you will experience a euphoric mood interspersed with bursts of unmotivated laughter . . . There is no hangover or harmful effect. On the contrary, a pleasant psychedelic afterglow appears quite regularly and may last several hours to several days.[6]

I looked at the preparation notes Natasja had provided:

> This is most significantly a holistic reset that allows for a deep release of destructive emotional and mental patterns, as well as an influx of life force that is both inspirational and healing . . . This is not a recreational drug and is certainly not for everybody.

Being forced to let go of the ego is precisely what draws many people to *Bufo*. The dissolution experience can impart an understanding and acceptance of mortality that helps to overcome the fear of death. It can also break attachments with past trauma, negative behaviours, and habitual negative thought patterns.

Natasja had written a chapter for a book called *Psychedelics and Psychotherapy: The healing potential of expanded states.* Her chapter, entitled, 'The Deep Dive into *Bufo alvarius* (5-MeO-DMT)' provides a breakdown of what she has observed as a facilitator on retreats:

> I have witnessed about a quarter of participants experience an ineffable sense of divine bliss and love with Bufo. Another quarter experience facing and processing their emotional blockages and traumas. The remainder have a range of

experiences, often transcending identity and duality but with a more neutral emotional tone. A few people return with no recollection of the journey at all.[7]

So, some people completely forget what happens. I was worried that I'd be one of them given that I'd blacked out, or dissociated, for two or three hours in one of my psilocybin trips. I didn't want to travel across the world for an experience that I was not even present for. I was grateful there would be two ceremonies—surely, I wouldn't forget both of them.

Rejection sensitivity

For the next retreat, I would again need an intention, and trying to come up with one plunged me into my usual indecision. After hours of walking and talking with Luke, I settled on addressing what my psychology textbooks had called 'rejection sensitivity'. It's part of a normal life to lose contact with friends or to outgrow each other, yet it always left me ruminating for years every time it happened. I'd reminded myself numerous times, over the years, of the adage that 'friends come into our life for a reason, a season or a lifetime' yet my internal monologue can sound like, 'What did I do wrong? Was it the time I said X, or the day I did Y? Is there something wrong with me that I can't see, some kind of dreadful blind spot? What, oh what, turned her off me? How could she just dump me out of the blue?'

The first time I ever lost a close friend, back in my twenties, I ruminated on it obsessively and even had numerous nightmares about the loss. Was it a simple matter that this experience had worn a deep groove in my brain for the future so that the slightest rejection sent me falling back into this well-worn neural pathway? The ridiculous part was that often I was in complete agreement that a friendship had run its course, but I still dwelt on the pain of rejection.

The first COVID lockdown brought the end of my marriage but also a loss of friends. When a marriage breaks down, it's common to lose friends as people take sides, but that didn't happen for me as most of my friends were not Marek's. Still, when you are suddenly single among long-term couples, and maybe even out there dating as I was, you become 'different' or 'other' for some. Humans have evolved to befriend those similar to themselves. The similar, the known, has been less of a threat to survival. These days, this may all happen at a subconscious level as humans get on with doing what humans do: cultivating friendships with people just like them.

It's not that I'm a needy person: I love, and need, solitude. I experience more JOMO (Joy of Missing Out) than FOMO. On reflection, the part that hurts is feeling uncared for—we all want to feel like there are people who have our backs or who have compassion for us in hard times. The rejections I've experienced have left me hurt by the lack of concern for my feelings. Yet, what do I expect, really? People are never going to sit down and list the things they don't like about you before wishing you a nice life—it's far easier to fade out of the picture with no explanations offered. So, despite the fact that mentally I can understand why the loss of friends happens, it still leaves me a ruminating wreck.

First group Zoom from Sydney

Despite the 4 a.m. start, I'd been looking forward to the first group Zoom meeting. I'd been too distracted to look forward to the retreat as I finished up all the loose ends of the final days in my job. I knew I'd start to grow excited once I turned my mind to preparing for the retreat and meeting the other participants.

Natasja opened, 'Well, it's nice to see my first balanced Bufo group: four women and four men—usually it's more like six men and two women for Bufo retreats.'

We all introduced ourselves, but a standout for me was Jimmy, who spoke with a strong New Zealand accent. He lived in Portugal, only a 45-minute drive from where the retreat would take place, with his beloved French-Portuguese wife and their one-year-old son. He was an open book: born on the sleepy South Island of New Zealand, he lost his mother at five years old when she died. His father then took a mining job and moved to Papua New Guinea, taking Jimmy and his brother. He described his upbringing as 'dysfunctional' due to his father's alcoholism. He hoped that on this retreat he might be able to 'let go of the pain of the past'.

Nobody in this group was new to psychedelics as between them they had attended ayahuasca retreats, experienced all that LSD has to offer or attended Natasja's previous retreats. The strange point of commonality was that almost all of us were between jobs, on the brink of starting a new career adventure. Natasja said it was common for there to be patterns of similarity in each retreat group. Two of us came from Australia, a couple from Russia, two from England and Jimmy from down the road but originally New Zealand.

Natasja introduced the two space holders who'd help her on the retreat: Sandra, an Austrian yoga teacher and breathwork specialist, and Jessica an experienced retreat facilitator. Sandra lived with her Italian partner in Austria but was keen to move to Portugal. She had a background hosting breathwork retreats and classes[8] and she'd set up an animal shelter in Greece for abandoned dogs, into which she poured a large part of her earnings. Born in the United States, Jessica helped facilitate, on average, 24 retreats a year. With a masters in Chinese medicine, she'd also run acupuncture practices in several cities of the world, including New York.

The diet would be slightly easier than for the psilocybin retreat and would only apply to the four days prior rather than the whole week, although Natasja encouraged us to do more than the four days if we could: 'no sugar, no salt, no red meat, no caffeine, no alcohol, no sex, no masturbation, avoid television'. Most difficult of all for me, was the rule of no other drugs which would mean giving up the CBD and THC that had cured my insomnia. There would be some long days ahead without caffeine to revive me after a restless night, but at least I'd be in the vibrant city of Lisbon.

One email from Natasja, following the Zoom, had encouraged something . . . odd:

> This may feel odd at first, but it can be incredibly helpful to start a conversation with the spirit of the medicine, the Toad. Speak to the Spirit and tell it your intentions. Tell

> it that you are coming to join in the ceremony. Ask for gentle lessons if that is what you need. Having a personal relationship with the medicine will make the experience of them in your body during the ceremony more comfortable. Remember that these medicines have spirits and that we are engaging with their wisdom with respect.

To my surprise, speaking at points throughout the day to the toad started to feel quite natural.

Arrival in Portugal

After three flights, which took 33 hours including layovers, I was finally in Lisbon, Portugal. It had been over 30 years since I'd last been there, and I had fond memories from when I visited as a 22-year-old. I could still remember my *Let's Go!* guidebook had described Lisbon as 'grimy but stately, shabby but alluring'. The description had amused my little travel group of school friends, and we would exclaim this quotation many times a day as we surveyed the charming streets.

Lisbon is just so damn appealing, helped by being the warmest city in Europe and by the sheer number of its attractions. Packed with charisma, in many ways it's a mini-Paris with similar architectural features: a Champs-Elysees equivalent, an Arc de Triomphe equivalent, a River Seine equivalent and town squares in the French style. After a devastating earthquake in 1755, the rebuild had been informed by the principles of the French Age of Enlightenment.[9] With its diverse history, Moorish and Roman architectural influences both abound.

Walking those narrow, cobblestoned streets, there was a surprise around every corner—with its steep hills it's common to discover a stunning view between buildings or to suddenly find yourself at a lookout, or you might get a glimpse of the river, or discover that you've inadvertently found your way back to where you started.

The Portuguese have no qualms about unconventional colours: buildings are often in pastel shades of baby blue, spearmint green, or musk pink, or covered in their classic blue-and-white tiles with pictures glorifying national heroes, battles or religious icons. I could've wandered those streets and alleyways for far more days than the five I had allotted as my reward for surviving the flight.

The retreat would take place on the Algarve, or the southern coast, that mecca for English and German retirees attracted by the sunshine and stunning coastline of sandstone cliffs and cave networks. I was saving the Algarve for after the retreat.

Zoom with Natasja

Natasja had organised a one-to-one Zoom with each retreatant as part of the preparation for the retreat. I fired up my computer from the kitchen benchtop of my tiny Airbnb studio apartment.

'What are the chances that I'll be one of those people who just forget the whole thing?' I asked her.

'About 50 per cent,' Natasja laughed. 'But don't worry about that, the days after you take the medicine can be where it all starts happening.'

'I can't stop thinking of Michael Pollan describing it as "just horrible". Could it be the same for me?'

'Anything can happen, but try to trust, with good set and setting, we get an experience that can teach us something valuable. Even difficult journeys can be really useful in the long run.'

'The more I look into this medicine the less I feel I know what to expect,' I lamented.

'Well, Bufo provides an open and ambiguous experience. It's an unstructured space with fewer things like the deities you meet with regular DMT, but something might get unlocked. It's more a feeling state than a knowing state. It's physical and psychological, not cerebral. It might not even make sense at first, but you may be able to impose a structure on what happened further down the track.'

Funny that Natasja mentioned meeting deities. Months before taking Bufo there had been an entity, of sorts, lurking in my consciousness, one I had seen in a painting. On a stopover in Tokyo, I'd visited an art gallery where I saw a painting of the Buddhist Goddess of compassion, Kuan Yin, standing on the head of a dragon in rough seas, one hand raised as if to say 'stop'. I was struck by the sheer feminine power of the painting and snapped a photo with my phone. Back in Sydney, the painting kept popping up in my consciousness at random moments throughout the day. It wasn't that I knew the first thing about Kuan Yin—deities were never the slightest part of my Buddhist practice as a 'rational Westerner'. Soon I began to wonder if maybe I'd meet Kuan Yin when I took Bufo, but encounters with deities were more likely on regular DMT and not 5-MeO-DMT—the other name for Bufo—that I was about to take.

'I see your intention,' Natasja changed the subject, 'will be around what you call your rejection sensitivity?'

'Yes, I guess because my mind still ruminates on friends I've lost over COVID. I feel like the more I lose friends the less social confidence I have—even at work. It makes me paranoid, as I worry people are seeing something in me that I can't.'

'Have you ever considered looking at it from an intergenerational trauma perspective?' Natasja asked. 'Trauma is stored in our DNA and when you experience relationship traumas it amplifies those that you carry from your parents, grandparents and even your ancestors. Then again, you might have a core belief, such as 'nobody cares about me' or 'I'm unlovable', and you only see the confirming evidence and nothing else. It's like a pregnant woman notices all the pregnant women. But let's try and put your intention in positive language. Instead of "deal with rejection sensitivity", what's an affirming belief you can work towards?'

After some back and forth, we came up with: 'I will find the social self-confidence to connect with others from a place of love.'

6

Bufo in Portugal

I WAS THE FIRST to arrive at Faro Airport, on the south coast of Portugal, from where a van would collect us. Meeting each retreatant face-to-face was the usual reminder that what people look like on Zoom rarely correlates with how they present in person. Riding in the van, I instantly bonded with Sam from England given both of us had recently attended one of Natasja's psilocybin retreats. Sam could barely contain her excitement, an excitement she shared with her husband back home, about the power of psychedelics, which she believed had changed her life in numerous, profound ways. At various points throughout the retreat she'd proclaim, 'We need to all play a part in *normalising* these medicines to others so they can help more people.' Despite carrying some heavy emotional burdens in her daily life, on the retreat she never stopped smiling.

Natasja, Danielle the chef and the two space holders, Jessica and Sandra, stood at the door of a country home to greet us. In character with so much of Portugal, the house was charming and full of character with a natural beauty that had no need for modern gloss and luxury. White stucco walls with a terracotta roof, it had an open plan on a single level, featuring a long dining table. The property was in a remote location and boasted a small swimming pool, a pond full of carp and a couple of teepees for ceremonies. Perched on a mountaintop, it overlooked rolling hills sprinkled with multicoloured wildflowers. Even the natural landscape of Portugal keeps with the description of charm over shine. Nature had a scrubby, scraggly quality due to a lack of rain, and the stunning wildflowers were more hardy than pretty. Many compare the landscape to Australia where the dryness, in places, precludes any deep greens, but still allows for beauty.

We all assembled in the 'yoga room' where Natasja welcomed us and gifted us all with a bottle of calming Bach flowers, made from wild plant extracts, to drop under our tongues throughout the retreat. She explained that each day would end with a plant bath where we would pour a jug of hot water and plant choppings over our bodies and dry ourselves by air, not towel, so that the flowers could work their magic on us overnight.

We then had time to settle into our rooms and I was delighted to be sharing with Sam. We would sleep in one of a series of newly built tiny houses in which our bedrooms were separated by a bathroom. Each house had a deck out the front where we could sit and gaze out over the hills that seemed to reach the horizon. From the moment I arrived, in April 2023, the sun shone down faithfully, and every day was around 23 degrees.

I loved mealtimes, not just for the nourishing, locally grown food, but for the chance to get to know the other retreatants. Jimmy from New Zealand continued to harness my attention with his willingness to trust the group and be vulnerable. I've given him the name Jimmy as he reminded me of Australian rock icon Jimmy Barnes. Like the singer, Jimmy had been the lead singer in a hard-rock band, he had the tattoos, the motorbikes, the 'dysfunctional family background' and the alcohol problem. He'd start weeping after every session and feel embarrassed, unaware of how it only made the group love him more. His intention for the retreat was 'to let go of the pain of the past', but also to conquer his alcohol addiction, which he defined as a difficulty stopping at one drink.

Rapeh and first breathwork

Seated in a circle in the teepee, Natasja introduced *rapeh*:

> Rapeh carries the spirit of the Grandfather Mapacho—Mapacho being the name of the tobacco plant—who is connected to all the other plant spirits. In just one blow into your nose, rapeh takes you out of your head and into your heart to connect with your essence. It cleans your energy field, removes blockages and sharpens your mind. It creates a sacred moment with you and your spirit.

Rapeh is tobacco that is blown up your nose using an applicator called a *tepi*. A ceremonial medicine, used throughout the Americas for thousands of years, it's a healthy and deeply spiritual way of ingesting tobacco. Highly respected as a medicine, it's deemed the 'master plant teacher', and is still used throughout the Amazon today for healing physical and spiritual ills.

Now it was my turn for Sandra to blow the rapeh up each of my nostrils.

Highly unpleasant as it enters your nose, rapeh made me feel still, present—and then amazed at how still and present I could be. My monkey mind stopped for several minutes as I was at one with myself, just me. Only three things existed: darkness, the breath and me, with my stilled mind, just sitting there, unperturbed by anything.

It wore off in no time and Sandra introduced our breathwork session.

We lay on our backs. Sandra provided some simple breathing instructions and started the powerful music.

My stomach clenches hard. Marek's face appears. Oh God, not Marek again. Didn't I finish with you back on the psilocybin retreat? I have a flashback to the moment we stood across the room from each other, some months after our split, in our empty, cleaned-out family home, the new owners about to move in the next day, and we both hugged our last hug in that house. I receive another image of Marek as my baby, nestled in my arms, and I realise we've known each other through many lifetimes.

Then the spirits of my sons join Marek and mine and I see that we've all been learning from each other over the lifetimes. Our faces form a whirl, and we all fuse into one and I feel love but sense the message: now spread this love to others.

In the sharing circle afterwards, I blurted to the group: 'I had this vision and realised my ex-husband and my sons and I have known each other over many lifetimes and that solves the mystery of why I still feel such a strong bond with my ex.'

I had imposter syndrome—I sounded like a believer in reincarnation, but I wasn't. Nor am I a disbeliever, though. Moreover, this breathwork ceremony lacked what some in the psychedelic world call 'noetic quality'. That is to say, it lacked authority or gravitas. I did not have the 'wow' or the certainty that comes with a deeply felt insight. I wasn't completely sure I hadn't made it all up. It felt like I was slowly warming to the idea of reincarnation but wasn't there yet. It had never been a concept that any of my Buddhist teachers, all from the West, gave any airspace.

One reason the idea of reincarnation appealed to me was that it explained how I feel about Marek: a strong, unbreakable bond. I care deeply for his wellbeing, and we would both do anything for each other, but why did I feel this way? When internet dating—and I had eleven dates before I met Luke—everyone without exception had a hostile relationship with their ex-partner. I was told that was the norm. Marek and I, like many couples together for decades, could certainly find some reasons to despise each other but we had managed to let bygones be bygones and maintained a close friendship, even since he'd moved back to Poland and re-partnered. It was a puzzle to me that I felt the way I did, and I felt that reincarnation was a possible explanation: maybe we'd known each other through many lifetimes and been each other's mother, brother, friend or partner?

Then again, there's a chance that the spirits had just set me up to help someone else, as Jimmy would, the next day, give me a hug and whisper in my ear: 'I can't stop thinking about what you said yesterday after the breathwork, and it's helped me. A lot.'

The setting for Bufo

We assembled as a group for Natasja to provide our orientation. 'Many of you will have participated in other retreats where we all took the medicine at the same time and sat together while the medicine took effect. With Bufo each of you will take the medicine separately. Bufo comes on within seconds and is over within half an hour, maybe less, so it requires focused supervision on one person at a time. Only Sandra and I will be with you and when you're finished, you'll head to the group room. There, Jessica will receive you and help you start your integration. The ceremonies will all take place in the teepee.'

Most of our day would be spent waiting: for our own ceremony and then for the rest of the group to finish, a process that would take about nine hours for the hardworking facilitators and give the rest of us a lot of time on our own. I'd have to wait three hours before my turn, and I had precisely nothing to do. I decided to take a slow stroll around the grounds with my hands loosely clasped behind my back like an elderly lady, stopping occasionally to examine the wildflowers, listen to the buzz of the bees and appreciate the sunshine, while ignoring the occasional butterfly in my stomach regarding what was ahead.

First Bufo ceremony

I couldn't suppress the nervousness and neither could my flipping stomach. Pollan's words were circling, 'It was just horrible', along with a fear that there might be physical pain with a drug so strong.

Before entering the teepee, I stood up straight, arms out, for the smudging that I remembered from the psilocybin retreat where Sandra ran a burning smoky sage stick around the perimeter of my body.

It comes on in seconds. The boundaries of my body disappear as I become colours and shapes—the colours of the sandstone of the Algarve. My body has never felt so comfortable and beyond the reach of pain, utterly anaesthetised, as though injected with serenity. Like a bird, I fly over multiple scenes of ancient sandstone structures, castles and forts, orange walls with cracked paintwork.

But now I'm back in my body, which is shaking violently, strong spasms in my throat, but numb and anaesthetised. I'm aware of my whiney little mind issuing instructions: 'surrender', 'feel into your body', 'how am I ever going to remember all this afterwards?', 'this is about your body not your mind'—and I wish it would quieten down and let me have the experience. I'm even conscious that the group seems behind schedule, and I don't want to take any extra time. But now the shaking stops and a deep peace descends on me.

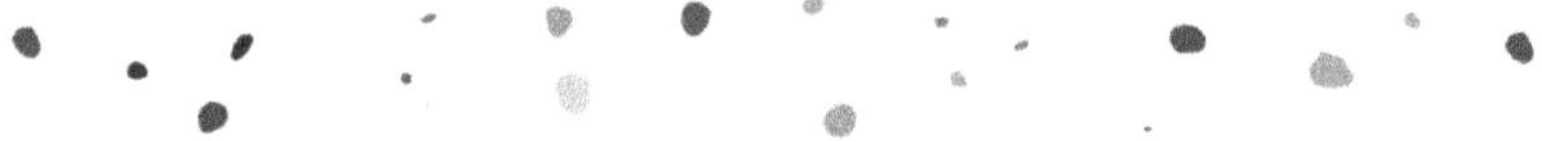

I opened my eyes to see Natasja and Sandra staring into my face.

'Hello, sleeping beauty,' Natajsa welcomed me back.

'I *wish*,' I replied, in some doubt that I looked beautiful.

'I could see your body calming down compared to yesterday in the breathwork. How do you feel?' asked Natasja.

'Serene,' I answered.

And that was all. Nothing whatsoever to be afraid of. The part of me I call the meaning-maker was somewhat disappointed, though: where is the message? Where is the takeaway? Something had definitely happened, but it felt too short to feel like more than a theme park ride. I remembered some of the images, but they didn't seem to have any particular significance. At least I would feel no fear for the Bufo ceremony tomorrow. As Natasja had told us, a first journey can be 'dipping your toe in the water' to test how it feels.

I was more than ready, and extremely relieved that there would be a second dive, but there was no denying it: I had wanted more to happen. I was worried I'd only feel underwhelmed by my Bufo journeys, but reminded myself that Natasja had told us many times that it's an ever-unfolding experience and the learning can happen days, weeks or months down the track if we take integration seriously. I had to have faith—never my strong point.

Integration with Jessica

I walked up a hill to be 'received' by space holder Jessica who would do a welfare check and decide whether I needed a blessing, a massage, some acupuncture or talking time. I left Jessica little choice as I started releasing my 'truth' all over her. I told her about my intention for the trip around rejection sensitivity and the pain I've felt from losing friends.

'I did read an article about that quite recently,' Jessica sympathised. 'It said that it can sometimes be even harder to lose a close friend than a partner. How is your relationship with yourself?' Jessica asked.

Perhaps a little raw after my trip, I disclosed to Jessica something I'd never told another human being. 'I think it's fine, these days, but a few years ago . . .' Here it came: 'I think I must've been depressed, and I struggled to sleep at night. I would lie in bed and imagine beating myself up. It was like I was divided into Bully-Sarah and Weak-Sarah. Bully-Sarah would kick Weak-Sarah hard, slam her into the wall, even hang her from a rope upside down by the ankle. Although I would never have acted on these fantasies, I still had a need to regularly run these violent visions through my mind.'

'What was going on in your life at the time?' Jessica asked.

'A bit of a cluster. I hated my job and the toxic politics there. I felt like I was failing at marriage, at friendships, at raising teenagers, but most painfully of all I felt uncared for, unloved, disconnected from the human race. It felt like I was dying of loneliness. My husband was an engineer, a pragmatist, a fixer and had no stock in trade with emotions that could not be put to any practical use, so I spared him from all knowledge of my mind-state. There were probably people that could've helped me, but I was voiceless to ask.'

'How have you been with self-compassion over the years?'

'I've practiced a lot of self-compassion, with success, but what bothered me, at that time, lying in my bed, was why I didn't inspire compassion in others? I'm in a good place now with all that and these days I do feel cared for, especially by my partner, but that was a time in my life when I didn't.'

I walked away feeling embarrassed. How could I have exposed all that? I'd never heard of anyone else fantasising about attacking themselves, although I did know of a mother who admitted to fantasies of packing her family into a car and crashing the car back and forth between two walls. Something she would, of course, never do, but the image helped her to vent. Jessica would have no personal experience of what I'd told her. With her natural blonde hair, blue eyes, bubbly conversation and hearty laugh, she was a people-magnet, easy to love. 'Surely such attractive people never feel rejected, or lonely, do they?' I sometimes catch myself lazily assuming.

I put the embarrassing disclosures behind me and spent the remaining hours, while the rest of the group had their ceremonies, by myself engaged in what some call 'mooching around'. My thoughts kept returning to what Danielle might cook for dinner—I was loving her vegetarian nourishment. I reflected on my ceremony, journalled a little, meditated sporadically.

When I least expected it, that dark part of my life with the self-harm fantasies would come up again.

Reviewing my first Bufo journey

By nightfall, in the closing circle after the first Bufo ceremony, Natasja advised us not to compare our experience with others, but nothing would stop me. As we went round the group, I heard the excitement in the voices as I caught the phrases, 'I died into the cosmos', 'I travelled through multiple universes', 'I accessed a higher consciousness'. I had done none of these things and started worrying that Bufo was not going to work for me. I eventually discovered that two other women in the group had felt a little underwhelmed, as I had, but, unlike me, one of them had been given a small dose. I felt like I'd been on a theme park ride, which was great, but I couldn't help asking, 'So what? How's that going to change my life?'. But at least I'd conquered any fear of Bufo and I knew I'd bring no fear into my next dive.

I couldn't believe that even during the trip, I was conscious of the ceremonies being behind schedule and the need to rush so that everyone else could have their turn. I don't know why I made this my problem, but it shows the importance of set, or mindset. Psychedelics are amplifiers and if you take any worries in, they may appear in an exaggerated form or hinder your capacity to surrender.

The next day I lay awake from 4 a.m. feeling flat that my first Bufo experience had not been 'bigger', but at 8 a.m. Sandra ran a powerful yoga session that left me raring to go for round two.

7

Second Bufo ceremony

We started in the yoga room with the usual passing of the talking stick round the group to share our internal weather. Just like me, everyone was buzzing after Sandra's powerful yoga session and full of anticipation for the ceremony ahead. Natasja began: 'Today's ceremony will be a little different from yesterday's as we'll all stay together and hold space for each other. We'll still go one by one but the whole group will be present for each journey in a support role. This is a chance for you to experience what it is to be a space holder, and I've had feedback in past retreats that it not only binds the group strongly but gives rise to more compassion for each other. It's a sacred experience to share.

'It won't be in the teepee today but outside, in nature, so bring your hats and sunscreen. Keep in mind for later at dinner, try to refrain from reflecting back to people what you observed about them during their ceremony. People may still be processing what happened. Besides, whatever they seemed to experience from an onlooker's perspective is unlikely to be what they actually experienced. You are likely only to see a projection of your own inner world onto another.'

An hour later, we all reassembled to sit on the grass, in the shade of a leafy tree.

For me, it was a day of the Buddhist practice of sending feelings of lovingkindness to each retreatant as they took the medicine. Every now and then I caught myself slipping into voyeur-mode, curious to watch other people's journeys, but I'd catch myself and return to the space-holding role.

The second trip

Sandra blessed me with the burning sage, and I sat on the blanket with Natasja and Sandra on either side of me, the group in a circle around us. I inhaled the Bufo deep into my lungs and held it a few moments.

It takes seconds, and my body starts to shake violently. I see rounded shapes the colours of watermelon and rockmelon, light oranges, soft reds, with rounded edges, billowing and circling over the top of each other. The contours of my body dance as I feel inflated and suffused with bliss. I squeeze my leg to check it's still there and it feels like reaching into a soft pillow. A strong cramp arises in my right leg, and I can see the cramp: concentric circles of bright colours, shaped like a lake. I surrender to the pain and let it do its worst. I breathe into it knowing, deeply, that I'm strong enough to bear it.

I see a large sign, 'PAIN IS MY TEACHER'.

But now I hover over myself lying in bed back in the family home, depressed. I'm in the period when I had the nightly fantasies of beating myself up. I burst into tears and hear Natasja, beside me, make a consoling noise. I was such a sad, alone figure and I ask, 'Why did it have to be so hard? Why wasn't anyone there for me?'

Suddenly I see random words float across my consciousness, 'You poor bastard', and I burst out laughing.

Then it hits me: I will write about this! I will become the Minister for Loneliness . . . an Ambassador for Loneliness. I'm not on this Earth to be the happy-go-lucky type, I have important things to do. Now hang on a sec, I'm being ridiculous, this is ego inflation. Still, stop being ashamed of that loneliness. There's a loneliness epidemic out there. Write about it.

The peak of the trip passes, and two memories arise: the time I stood in the Buddhist library reading the back of a book and felt a rush of love hit me. I'd felt, with utmost certainty, that someone had just sent me lovingkindness. The second memory is a Buddhist teacher on a stage in a crowded marquee comforting a crying woman who begged for answers. It was one of those problems to which there were no answers and I wondered what on earth the teacher would say. She said, 'Do you believe there's enough love in this room to contain your pain?' The woman nodded as the teacher placed a loving hand on her back to channel the love.

Out of nowhere Luke's smiling face zooms towards me. We embrace in a heavenly hug, our two bodies swirling fast into a blur until we become one.

I opened my eyes. Natasja asked, 'Can you give us a sense of how you feel?'

'I feel a sense of purpose.'

As the minutes after the trip became hours, I grew worried. Only a day ago I'd told Jessica my biggest secret, which became the focus of my trip. I had no choice but to write about that very secret in my book, something I had no desire to do. While I may seem like a happy over-sharer, I do have my secrets. Then again, maybe the toad had a point and there was a bigger picture to consider than my poor little ego.

I was also confused by the message 'PAIN IS MY TEACHER'. It sounded like some corny cliché with no immediate relevance. Or was this a message to pass on to my son Alex who had lived with chronic pain for years from sports injuries? Maybe it would be useful for the many hours of dental work facing me on my return to Australia.

I even had some niggles about the power of love as it appeared, after the peak of my trip, in the Buddhist library and with the Buddhist teacher in the marquee. Don't people need love from real human beings rather than an anonymous person in a library or, as that teacher suggested 'everyone in the room'? It would take several psychedelic trips for me to understand that love doesn't always need to come from another person—it's out there, and within us all for the taking if we choose to avail ourselves of it.

I noticed that I seemed to be caught in heady meaning-making, when maybe the real journey was for my emotions and body sensations.

The final ceremony, a breathwork ceremony the next day, would answer most of these questions.

Cacao ceremony

For the cacao ceremony the following day, a new facilitator, Mela, joined the retreat for the afternoon. This ceremony would take place outside on a patch of ground with a picturesque view of the hilltops below. We assembled in the shade as the sun shone brightly from a cloudless blue sky. A light, cool breeze lingered, so conditions were ripe for magic.

Mela introduced herself by sharing the story of her adult life, a journey from feeling lost and alienated in her early twenties to finding her voice, and her calling, with the passing years. Openly revealing her vulnerabilities, Mela created a space for deep sharing. One by one, we approached her to ladle some thick, dark cacao into a mug, which we all glugged down while she asked each of us, one after another, to come forward to say our prayer to the spirit of cacao. I spoke aloud my intention for the retreat: to feel calm and confident with others, for my ego-protective tendencies to get out of the way so I could connect lovingly.

From that point, Mela arranged a series of games which, with the help of the cacao, made me feel like a happy, giggly little girl. The afternoon felt like a return to the best of childhood. We all lost our inhibitions and engaged fully in playful activities. In one moment, we were decorating each other's faces with face paints, the next we competed to produce the silliest laugh. A dance interlude turned into a round of go-into-the-middle-of-the circle-and-do-something-silly-for-the-group-to-imitate.

Finally, the most touching activity was for each group member to have a turn sitting in the chair while the others stood around showering that person with praise—an activity filled with as many warm moments as hilarious ones, as we all came in close and patted, stroked or whispered into the ear of the person in the hot seat: everything from, 'You always exude warmth and joy' to, 'You've got really nice clothes'. Some group members wept during their turn in the chair, which further opened our hearts for each other.

By the end of the cacao ceremony, I was amazed at how happy I'd felt. I hadn't been this happy since . . . maybe the cacao ceremony on the psilocybin retreat when I had also felt connected back to childhood joy through drawing with coloured pencils, through dancing and group sharing of our deepest desires for our lives.

Unfortunately, the strong dose of cacao meant that I would not sleep that entire night. I wish that was the only twist in the tail but, in addition, Natasja had been unable to join us in the cacao ceremony amid murmurings that she was attending to some plumbing issues. Sam and I had failed to listen to the instruction that the toilets in the tiny houses would not accept toilet paper, which needed to be stowed in the bin beside the toilet. So while I was at the cacao ceremony having the time of my life (literally), Natasja was stuck dealing with all my shit (literally).

Straight after the cacao ceremony we filed into the yoga room where Mela ran our second breathwork ceremony. I had zero expectations for the session as I was yet to experience a strong insight, or a major breakthrough, in a breath session. Boy was I in for a surprise.

Breathwork ceremony

I hope I'm doing this right . . . nothing seems to be happening . . . here comes my usual spasming and trembling and clenching in the guts but hang on, what is that tingling in my hands? Actually, it's more than just tingling, they feel like they're being jack-hammered, they shake as though battery-operated. My thighs join in . . . something has taken possession of me. The boundaries of my body dissolve and I'm back to feeling like a mass of billowy cushions as though yesterday's Bufo trip is continuing.

Something, a powerful spiritual force of intense tightening, slowly works its way up my body. It brings painful cramps, but I know, deeply, that it will move through my body and leave me with a sense of deep peace. I just need to breathe into the pain and allow it to be there. I've got this. This pain will not overpower me. The cramps are strong in the same place as yesterday: my right buttock and thigh and then my wrist—the same wrist cramps I experienced in my psilocybin retreat. This is fun, though—something spiritual, supercharged and mysterious is unfolding.

I receive a stream of insights. The toad, the plants. They will handle my writing project. Just trust them. They'll speak through me. Share everything from my trips. People need to hear my struggles. Don't be precious. They'll understand. Stop protecting your ego.

The force has now made its way through my body, and I'm left with a deep sense of peace, as I knew I would be. My eyes shut, I'm aware of the two space holders at either side of me, tightly holding an upper arm with one hand, and my hand with their other. But why would they be so focused on me when there are several others in the room? Why do I get so much of their time? But now I realise they aren't there at all, and I see that it's Kuan Yin. Two Kuan Yins sit on either side of me as we three commune together in a grassy meadow bathed in sunshine, surrounded by wildflowers.

I focus on my hands, which feel like swollen baseball mitts and marvel that I can feel so vividly the sensations of a hand in mine, in both of mine. I concentrate on these sensations in amazement—little has ever felt more real than these hands in mine. I stay with the sensations and then realise there is a Kuan Yin at each of my feet. Four Kuan Yins, all sitting calmly as they convey peace and serenity and even amusement at the situation. I know the unspoken message is, 'You are loved, Sarah'. I weep quietly and want to stay here endlessly . . .

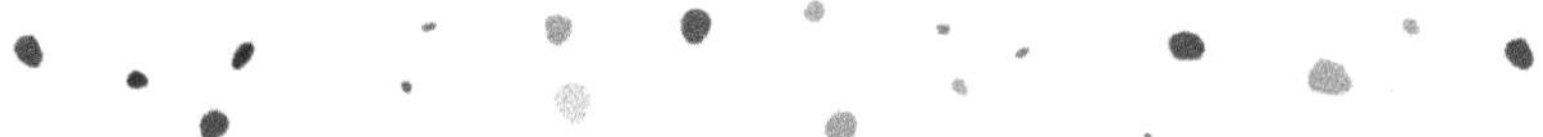

Mela encouraged us to sit up and return to the group. I processed my momentary disappointment that I must leave the Kuan Yins but sat in a state of wonderment as we share in the group.

'I just had the most amazing experience of my life,' I enthused. 'It was like some kind of cosmic joke. An experience I'd hoped for happened four times!'

I loved that Kuan Yin, just like in the painting, had spared me any eye contact or any saintly smile. Her loving presence was quiet, dignified and far more powerful than any facial expression could convey.

The rest of the group was similarly enthusiastic, particularly Sam who described her experience: 'I have so much mother guilt to process, but I had a vision of myself lying in a bed as an elderly woman with my two adult sons standing at my bedside showering me with compliments about what a fabulous mother I'd been. It was so moving, and it's made me feel like I may be doing a much better job as a mother than I've ever believed.'

Jimmy said, 'I've stopped crying. There are no more tears left. The pain has gone.'

I later asked Natasja: 'That breathwork session was the strongest trip I've had on the retreat. What was it? The breathwork? The cacao? Yesterday's Bufo? A combination of all of them?'

'I'd say the combination of all of them,' she answered.

Closing session

Day five, the final day, and Jessica treated us all to an acupuncture session. The edge comes off the achiness from my fully sleepless night as I enjoyed a subtle bodily thrum from the needles.

Natasja provided some advice for our integration over the coming weeks.

'The first thing for us all to note about any medicine journey is that a ceremony will not magically fix all our problems. That's *our* work, the integration work, when we grow into a new way of being. So how do you do that work?

'Try your best to make time for rest and reflection and, if at all possible, avoid being swept up in too much busyness. We all need a self-care practice to make the best of the window of neuroplasticity in our brains that the medicine opens.

'Choose activities that support the integration such as creative pursuits—art, dance, journalling or embodied activities like yoga, breathwork, acupuncture or time in nature.'

'Compared to how I felt after psilocybin,' an English woman asked, 'the Bufo experience is already feeling a little distant. Is there a way to make it feel closer?'

'Be attuned to what emotions arise for you. What are you feeling and where do you feel it in your body? Meditation is an excellent integration tool. If you find unpleasant emotions arise, make space for them rather than resist them. Create a compassionate and accepting container for anything to arise.'

'Do you think there is any role for the thinking mind?' I asked. 'I know the body and the emotions are probably better teachers, but I can't turn my analytical mind off.'

'I'd say, don't rush into making meaning and trying to interpret sessions,' Natasja replied. 'If you make space in your life, it will all unfold at a natural pace. You've started a process that unfurls over the days, weeks and months and not just during the ceremony. I do encourage people to speak to a therapist, or a close friend, but don't treat that as an excuse to go back into your head. We do need to connect to others as we integrate, and share what we learn by talking, but as you do so, be aware of your body sensations and emotions—you may even find that sometimes they don't support your words, and that can be something to explore.'

8

Reflecting on the Bufo retreat

I'M BACK IN SYDNEY, two weeks after the retreat, on a one-to-one Zoom with Natasja.

'You mentioned, I remember, after the breathwork session, a cosmic joke?' Natasja asked.

I told Natasja how I'd expected no deities on Bufo, given that it was more likely on regular DMT, but I'd still thought it would be exciting to meet Kuan Yin. To see her four times in the one vision made me feel like something out there really loved me.

'Thanks so much for telling me that,' she began. 'I'd felt Kuan Yin's presence when I did the opening for the second Bufo ceremony and I'd wondered who she was there for—now I know.'

'Is that true?' I asked in disbelief.

'Don't you remember, I acknowledged the presence of Kuan Yin as part of my opening for the group?'

'Come to think of it, I remember that clearly now,' I replied. 'It had slipped my mind what with so much going on.'

'Yes, I always acknowledge the members of the group in my opening of the ceremony and then I tune in to who else might be present and I definitely sensed the presence of Kuan Yin—that's why I named her to the group.'

'Too amazing,' I replied. 'And speaking of things that are a bit out there, I seem to be in regular conversation with the giant toad in my mind. Remember in the first email you sent us you told us to start developing a relationship with the spirit of the medicine? The toad? So now I'm not a God-botherer but a toad-botherer. If I'd known six months ago that I'd be praying to a toad, I would've been a little concerned.'

'I understand that talking to a spirit animal might feel unusual,' Natasja replied, then grinned broadly, 'but really, nobody knows shit about what's out there.'

'I just find myself throughout the day saying things like "Thanks for that, Toad" or, "Please help that suffering person, Toad" or, "Please let me fall asleep, Toad". Should I stop this now and go back to normal?' I asked.

'As long as you don't give away your power. Hold on to your sovereignty. But on another note, tell me how things went with your intention.'

'Oh yeah, with my so-called rejection sensitivity. I guess, when I think about the handful of friends I lost over COVID, the drama seems a little more distant. Like, before the retreat my thoughts about losing them felt quite immediate whereas now that loss feels like something that happened many years ago. I'm definitely ruminating less.'

'And how about the commitments we each made on the retreat to help us integrate things into our daily lives?'

'Yes, I made a commitment to do daily lovingkindness meditation where I send out feelings of love to a variety of people. I feel like that's the best way to achieve my intention of connecting with others more lovingly and to ensure my interactions are less about me and my insecurities.'

'Great! So, is there anything else you wanted to raise about your integration?'

'There's one thing that falls into the category of a miracle, or a healing, or a miraculous healing. Have you heard of sciatica?'

'I haven't,' Natasja replied.

'I don't have a diagnosis,' I explained, 'but I think I've had a condition called sciatica where I get strong pain going from my right buttock down the back of my thigh, but only when I sit for a long time. I've had it for years but it's manageable if I avoid sitting for too long. It's meant that I have to take lots of breaks at work to stretch my right leg and it makes travelling, in cars, on public transport and especially on the flight to Europe, very challenging—sometimes I have to stand up for hours on a flight as my leg hurts so much.'

Natasja managed not to glaze over as I banged on about my ailment.

'Well, in the second Bufo ceremony,' I continued, 'I spent probably half the trip bringing awareness to a cramp in my right leg, which I perceived as a lake of concentric circles of bright colours. I tried to breathe into it and allow the pain to exist. The same pain arose in the breathwork session too. Anyway, on the four-hour bus trip from the retreat to the airport I noticed I had no leg pain. I was amazed but knew the two flights ahead of me would be the real test. So, I got through the first flight, which was around eight hours and then I made it through the second flight, which was about thirteen hours. No leg pain. That felt like an utter miracle to me.'

'Well, time will tell, I guess,' replied Natasja.

'In that second Bufo trip the leg cramp happened right before I revisited a time in my life when I was depressed, so I'm guessing I stored the pain from that period of my life in my leg and the Bufo released it.'

'Maybe,' replied Natasja with a shrug. I love that she's happy to make space for mystery, or what Zen Buddhists would call 'not-knowing'.

On the subject of healing, on one of the two group Zooms after the retreat Jimmy told the group:

> Looking back, my issues got solved in a different way to what I expected. A big thing for me has always been my drive for self-destruction, but the infinite love I experienced from the Bufo was so powerful that it could replace that drive. I saw on my trips that, ultimately, we are all pure love and that this could replace my drive for destruction and there has been so much relief for me in this realisation. Yesterday I had a beer with a mate. One only—I just don't feel like getting smashed anymore. I've been feeling so grateful. Every day. All day.

Jimmy paused as if suddenly realising something. Then his face lit up, 'Wow, I didn't cry.'

Quitting sugar

In the lead-up to the Bufo retreat I'd exchanged some messages with Darren, who I'd met on the psilocybin retreat. Without my even asking, Darren had volunteered, 'Since the last retreat I haven't had any caffeine or alcohol and I used to have one or two drinks a day.'

I was impressed. Darren beat two habits. I was tempted to try and beat my main addiction, sugar, but something was stopping me from making it a formalised intention for the Bufo retreat. I'd tried to quit sugar many times before and had always failed. I'd forced myself to watch anti-sugar documentaries. I'd ploughed through books condemning it and these efforts worked for a while but when sugar finally made its way back into my life I made up for lost time. The floodgates opened and the extended binge would begin. I have long been obsessed with nutrition and its potential to improve my daily wellbeing. I put hours every week into preparing healthy meals yet I self-sabotaged all this effort with numerous treats on the side. Emotional eating like this helped me cope with the sad stories I encountered doing my job.

I'd toyed with the idea of quitting sugar and had told Luke prior to the retreat.

'Who knows, maybe after this retreat, and now that I've quit my job, I might give it up?' I suggested.

'I don't think so, darling,' Luke teased. 'You'll be working from home with the supermarket and all that temptation just downstairs.'

He had a point. Living directly above a supermarket turned that place into another room of our house, a second kitchen. Many a day, I visited twice as we were free from the need to plan our shops.

Often—okay, daily—one of us would come back with a wicked grin, a glint of the devil in our eye, and a treat.

'Well, it doesn't make it any easier,' I struck back at Luke, 'that I'm living with someone who can freely indulge in all the things I love with zero repercussions to his health'.

'What do you mean?' Luke asked, disingenuously.

'I mean your four coffees a day, wine from Wednesday through to Saturday, almost daily packets of chips and frequent chocolate bars.'

'Well why don't you give my approach a try?'

'I have,' I moaned, 'I just have a sensitive body that punishes me for the slightest slip.'

Take my sugar addiction, for instance. My dental bills were through the roof, my cholesterol remained well above the guideline and the sugary snacks made me feel slightly sick, bloated and regretful, every time I indulged. Yet there was one aspect of my diet that bothered me more than any of these drawbacks: I was sick of being pushed around by my cravings. I resented the real estate sugar took up in my brain. It would be way too boring to include my daily inner monologue in the body of this book but see Appendix 2 if you want to hear how tedious sugar addiction (or any addiction?) can be. I wanted to free up that mental space to use on higher concerns. If our thoughts make our worlds, as the Buddha taught, I had to reduce the influence of my inner sugar addict.

I'd resisted setting an intention about sugar before, and during, the retreat, thinking it would fail as it always had in the past, but now that the retreat was over, I thought I'd try a 'take it day-by-day, one day at a time-type approach' and see what happened. Read: no pressure. I wanted to use the window of neuroplasticity the Bufo had created to override old habits. After all, an academic called Pedro had visited our retreat for a few hours as part of his research into how Bufo can lead to healthier life practices.

In the early days after the retreat, whenever I saw a tempting treat, I'd quickly look away and avoid thinking about what it might taste like. I had a few days left in Portugal and it was hard to avoid Portuguese tarts, which were often warm from the oven (someone told me). My mouth watered if I dwelled for even a second on anything sweet, so avoidance was the only answer.

But within a few weeks, I noticed my life was no longer run by cravings. I'd stopped wasting my time in self-remonstration. I felt better, physically and psychologically, as I was no longer digesting unhealthy food and processing guilt. Yet I could never have reached this stage through mere rationalising. My addiction was way too strong for a rational approach, which I'd tried many times. I knew the medicine was responsible.

One hears stories, and I've met a few people who have told me, that after taking psychedelics they lose all desire for smoking or drinking alcohol or caffeine. Addictions, occasionally, evaporate. It wasn't like that for me. Ice-creams, pastries and chocolate never lost their appeal, but it appeared my willpower had increased. I'd allow myself a treat every few weeks but now I was strong enough to resist my former pattern of daily indulgences.

Months later

Ever since the Bufo retreat I'd been shaking, trembling and spasming, at various points in the day. My throat spasmed, my torso shook, my head wobbled back and forth, my stomach clenched. Initially, I'd interpreted this as a good sign—I was releasing tension, processing mysterious spiritual energy—but now it had gone too far. It was happening too often throughout a normal day: on waking, during meditation, all the time if I was tired, at random moments for no reason, and when I lay in bed at night. Luke found it unsettling. My thoughts fell into that human tendency to catastrophise. What if the shaking turned into an all-day thing that never stopped? What if it happened around other people, or in future professional settings? My inner hypochondriac sprang to life and I started feverishly googling: maybe it was early-onset Parkinsons, or a syndrome I discovered called dystonia or some other kind of neurological disease leading to death?

Eventually I landed on a study that would put my mind at ease. It would even provide a word for my experience.

'. . . a phenomenon known as "reactivations" (similar to "flashbacks") is a poorly understood and frequently reported phenomenon which appears associated with 5-MeO-DMT [Bufo] use.'[1]

A reactivation was defined as including 'perceptual, somatic, or emotional sensations that were first experienced during the acute psychedelic state'. My shaking fell into the 'somatic' category, meaning it related to my body. Reactivations, the study said, are most commonly experienced in the first week or two after a trip but could go on for weeks or months. In a sample of 344, a whopping 73 per cent had experienced reactivation in the weeks following their Bufo trip. Of those, 86 per cent claimed it was a pleasant experience, a further 10 per cent said it was neutral, which left 4 per cent who'd had distressing reactivations. I'd describe my own as 'neutral', although they could feel annoying at times. The study also found reactivations were more likely for those who were: female, older age and, for some mysterious reason, tertiary-educated.

Well, of course! Natasja had even warned us about 'reactivations' but I'd assumed, in my ignorance, she'd meant visual flashbacks.

I received a text from Luke as I sat at my desk:

> Darling, I was thinking we should go to doctors together to discuss your shaking with them.

Instead of 'no', I replied:

> You're so sweet.

Luke:

> Loved 'You're so sweet'.

You have to feel for Luke. When he first committed to me, I was a mild-mannered public servant. Today his home pulsates to the rhythms of tribal drumming, his girlfriend does this freaky shaking thing at random moments and all she talks about is psychedelics. He's very patient.

I recently met a woman socially who'd been through extreme grief, loss and trauma. She shared with me that at points in her recovery she'd find her body shaking and her teeth chattering, but she learned that this was not something to 'fix', rather it was helpful to her recovery. She sent me a link to an international organisation called TRE, which stands for Tension & Trauma Releasing Exercises. I did their online course where they train people to lie on the floor and activate their innate capacity to tremble and shake.

With trainers all over the world, 42 in Australia, I felt satisfied, once and for all, that my trembling and shaking were no reason to consult a medical professional.

What do I take away from my Bufo experience?

In the second Bufo ceremony I'd returned to a time in my life when I was lying in bed, depressed and overwhelmed. I believe my body has released the stored pain from that time, leaving me more buoyant, less encumbered with stuck-ness. Psychiatrist Dr Rick Strassman, a pioneering researcher whose work I cover in chapter 19, wrote that to recover from trauma we need to confront it head on, usually through a voluntary re-experiencing of the feelings associated with the trauma: 'By experiencing absolute loss of control in a safe and supportive situation, it might be possible to more fully contact, and thereby own and let go of, certain painful emotions.'

Stan Grof, the 'Godfather of LSD' research and inventor of Holotropic Breathwork, referred repeatedly to the body's 'inner healing mechanism'.

That said, the pain in my leg, the sciatica, which I believed had been miraculously cured, returned about three weeks after the retreat. This, of course, felt disappointing but at least it returned in a milder form. It would disappear once and for all, however, after I took MDMA a few months later, as though the release of the emotional pain stored in my leg was finally complete.

As for my lost friends, I continue to think of them from time to time, and even feel some pain, but I no longer ruminate or battle intrusive thoughts. At least, when such thoughts arise, there is less emotional pain and more acceptance than there used to be.

The memory of Kuan Yin continues to be a source of comfort when I'm trying to fall asleep, when I need a comforting image and when I practise lovingkindness meditation. One example is when I recently lay in the dentist's chair. I knew that the next few minutes—or who knew how long?—were going to hurt real bad. I was about to sacrifice a molar, which would be pulled out of its ancient resting place with a tool resembling pliers. An inner panic began; there was no escape. I needed a comforting thought, and fast. And there I was again. Lying in that field, surrounded by four serene and unflappable Kuan Yins, sitting peaceably at each hand and each foot. The image was comforting, and I soon acknowledged that the numbing up from all those needles really worked.

I continue to practise Buddhist lovingkindness meditation, also called in the Buddhist tradition the *metta bhavana* meditation where you cultivate love in turn for: 1) yourself, 2) someone you love, 3) a neutral person that you have no particular feelings about, 4) a difficult person, and 5) everybody in the world in ever-expanding circles.

For all sorts of reasons, many meditators 'hate' practising lovingkindness meditation and a quick google of the words 'hate' and 'metta bhavana' reveals an online course called 'Who Hates the *Metta Bhavana*?' I'd tended to neglect *metta bhavana* myself, with the excuse that it always made my mind wander, especially when I focused on a difficult person. I'm still prone to distraction today when I practise it, but I realise that it's too important to neglect given its power to shape my heart into a more loving one. After all, I notice the difference it makes to all my relationships. It makes me more understanding and less judgemental—even difficult people are still precious.

Of course, some of the benefits of any trip are subtle, or imperceptible, and I may never consciously understand them. A journeyer can simply feel inexplicably lighter, or happier, in their daily life and not know why. On both retreats, facilitators had reminded us to avoid becoming obsessed with meaning-making and to resist the temptation to ask that very question: what did I get out of it? A large part of the answer will be an eternal mystery. In Michael Pollan's second book about plant medicines, *This Is Your Mind on Plants*, a Westerner asked a young Navajo man for an explanation of something that happened during his trip only to be told: 'That is the problem with you whites. You always want to know everything. We just experience it.'[2]

I'm reminded of the emphasis in Buddhism to rely less on thinking to resolve, or heal, life's conundrums. Thinking too much can tie us in knots when what we really need is that spaciousness we find during meditation, during time in nature or when we feel deeply connected to our loved ones. At such times, the body's inner healing mechanism will do its work. No thinking, or effort, required.

Nine months after the retreat I emailed Jimmy in Portugal for permission to include his experience in this book, which he granted, adding this paragraph:

> In the year after my son was born, for some reason, when he was crying or upset, I would also feel very emotional and felt a lot of pain from the past, around the tragic death of my mother from suicide when I was a child. My main intention for the

retreat was that the experience might help relieve this pain and help me get back to balance. I also 'liked a drink' which was linked, however that was the secondary intention. The two Bufo experiences, and the whole experience overall at the retreat, with the amazing guides, was incredibly powerful. After visiting a realm of eternal love on the Bufo, I was filled with an immense love that I had never felt before. I'm grateful to say that I no longer feel the deep pain inside that came to the surface from my past. I'm no saint lol, but I'm living a happier and healthier lifestyle now and loving being a father.

9

Holotropic Breathwork in Sydney

A STRONG DOSE OF psychedelics will definitely alter your state of consciousness. It may also provide healing or a mystical experience. Yet psychedelics are not the only way to achieve such experiences.

Back in 1970, President Nixon commanded that all research funding into psychedelics stop as he feared the link between acid and resistance to the Vietnam war, and the rest of the world followed his lead. In response to this devastating blow to scientific progress, leading LSD researchers Stanislav Grof, and his wife Christina, switched to developing Holotropic Breathwork as an alternative way to experience non-ordinary states of consciousness and gain access to the unconscious mind. Today, many psychedelic retreats include Holotropic Breathwork on their program and occasionally one-day workshops take place in the community.

The power of the breath has been recognised as a way to alter consciousness for thousands of years, by ancient cultures as well as modern religions, albeit the more mystical strains. In their book *Holotropic Breathwork*, Stanislav and Christina write, 'Since earliest history, virtually every major psychospiritual system seeking to comprehend human nature has viewed breath as a crucial link between the material world, the human body, the psyche, and the spirit.'[1]

The Grofs argue that healing occurs through gaining access to the hidden parts of ourselves so that we can integrate them, or acknowledge and own them, and live a fuller, more emotionally honest life as a result. The word 'holotropic' comes from the combination of two Greek words that translate to 'moving towards wholeness', which suggests bringing together all the different parts of ourselves, the unattractive ones as much as the attractive.

A Holotropic Breathwork experience is unlikely to be as powerful as an LSD experience. After all, an LSD trip can last up to twelve hours whereas a breathwork session is more like 90 minutes. Still, the gentler and shorter-lasting experience is bound to suit seekers who may hesitate, for whatever reason, to use psychedelics. Luke was one such character and I was delighted, at least initially, when he agreed to attend a workshop with me.

I'd received an informative email about a workshop taking place in the Sydney suburb of Newtown.

> Our body is where we hold emotions, memories and stories that often we don't have words for. It is also where we can access our fullest potential for everything we desire in life.
>
> Through this transformative Breathwork journey with Lynsey Chan, you will be guided into a powerful

> experience, reaching altered states of consciousness in support of your healing and self-discovery. This style of breathwork is inspired by Holotropic Breathwork which was originally created by Stanislav Grof in the 60's. The technique was created to achieve psychedelic-like states without using psychedelic drugs. The Grofs believed the process of deep, self-exploration brought on by these altered states can bring healing and Holotropic Breathwork has been a tool for therapeutic healing ever since.
>
> Lynsey and Guests will offer a safe container for you to reconnect to your natural medicines, your breath to break through and let go of old stories, reach higher states of consciousness where peace, embodiment, reconnection, love, joy, personal power, ecstasy, clarity and flow all live.

As if that didn't tick enough boxes, the proceeds of the event would go to a fund to help people suffering mental illness to access the newly legal medicines psilocybin and MDMA, as part of 'psychedelic-assisted psychotherapy'.[2]

I wondered if much research had been conducted into how effective Holotropic Breathwork could be as a tool for healing. The Grofs admitted that it was not warmly received by the academic world, nor clinicians, but they put that down to scientists' traditional rejection of anything from the spiritual world.[3] Another explanation is that the Grofs were proponents of the need to process birth trauma, based on their observations of thousands of birth trauma experiences during LSD trips, but the academic establishment has never accepted that a human can remember their birth.

In one study from the year 2015, Danish academics found research to date was scarce and set out to test whether Holotropic Breathwork could have any effect on the development of self-awareness.[4] Twenty participants undertook four Holotropic Breathwork sessions. The study measured a wide range of attributes relating to self-awareness, and found participants experienced improvements in their temperament, that they felt more sociable and had lower levels of interpersonal distress. As the study put it, participants found it 'easier to let go of conflicts and struggles about control'. In short, their self-awareness increased especially in social contexts.

Of course, a sample size of twenty where eleven of them were experienced holotropic breathers can't be the last word on the healing power of Holotropic Breathwork, but I managed to find a study with 11,000 participants—and made a mental note to share the findings with Luke.

Lead-up to the breathwork ceremony

On our Saturday walk around the park, Luke and I discussed the upcoming workshop.

'Can you think of an intention to take into the session?' I asked Luke.

'I think you know what my intention is,' Luke answered, and indeed I knew. He had a problem with rumination about one persistent problem in his life and had long craved relief. 'How about you?' Luke asked.

'I've noticed myself becoming frustrated, even cranky, about time management. I always feel like my working day at home gets eaten into by all life's other demands. I stress over whether I'm productive enough and that detracts greatly from my mood and my capacity to enjoy my life as it is.'

'Isn't that something that came up in your past trips?' Luke asked.

'Wow, you remember,' I replied. 'I had insights that I could leave my book project to the universe—or the plants, the toad, the Divine—and stop trying to control and worry everything into place. I had insights about the absurdity of daily life and what a waste of energy it is to let things get to you. I guess my habit of rushing and getting frustrated that the day is slipping away is very deep-seated so it's still there.'

'You do seem to be happy with how the book's going whenever I ask you,' Luke added.

'Yes, I don't stress about the book. I think I've integrated the insight that it's all taken care of by something greater than me. It's mainly life admin—and all those 'shoulds' like exercise, phone calls, housework, medical appointments—that stops me working on the book.'

Not for the first time, a conversation in the lead-up shaped my mindset, or 'set', and would influence the journey the next day.

'I'm not sure about this,' Luke raised on the drive across town to the workshop.

'Don't say that,' I moaned. 'If you're not fully on board, I'll feel responsible and that'll affect my mindset.'

'I just have a feeling nothing will happen,' Luke teased, 'and I'll be lying there for three hours, breathing in and out, wishing I'd chosen something better to do on a Sunday morning.'

'I thought it'd be an opportunity to help you decide if you want to try psilocybin,' I offered. 'It'll give you a taste of what it's like to have a trip, except with breathwork you have control—you can stop following the breath instruction, or even stand up and walk out, if it gets too much. With a psychedelic you can't jump off the bus.'

'I guess I just have no idea what to expect,' Luke admitted.

'Well, you certainly don't have to worry about safety,' I began my information dump. 'I was reading someone's PhD thesis this week and they had data for 11,000 psychiatric patients from a community hospital, who had all done some Holotropic Breathwork sessions. They collected the data over twelve years and there wasn't a single adverse incident reported—and that was what you could call a vulnerable population.'[5]

'I'm not worried about the safety,' Luke replied. 'Just that I'll waste my Sunday.'

'Well, they investigated 400 of those patients more closely, and over 80 per cent of them had a "transpersonal" experience—which just means an experience that took them outside their normal ego structure—something trippy, or otherworldly, if you like. Anyway, the weekly holotropic sessions at this hospital were popular and always booked out.'

'We'll see, I guess,' Luke responded cheerfully.

The workshop

We arrived half an hour early and watched the participants register and file in to a community hall dominated by a large, golden Buddha statue at the front. High, sloping ceilings, vases of flower arrangements and three cheerful volunteers, buzzing around, ensured a pleasant setting. As usual, I'd pictured a group of about seven only to find numbers more like 70. Lynsey Chan, with a microphone wired around her head, and her volunteers, tiptoed between the yoga mats, asking people to move their mats closer to fit more people in, and Lynsey, with her warm smile and ready laugh, was the picture of warm reassurance and approachability. Demographically, women slightly outnumbered men but participants came from all ages over eighteen. There was no particular 'hippie vibe' and everyone looked down-to-earth in their comfortable clothes.

That there was only Lynsey and three helpers in a room of 70 breathers was no cause for concern given Holotropic Breathwork operates on Stanislav Grof's premise that it's not the facilitator that creates any personal growth but rather 'the innate healing intelligence of the client's own psyche'.[6] The Grofs use phrases like, 'the intrinsic wisdom of the body' or the 'innate healer' as they believe that non-ordinary states activate an 'inner radar that automatically finds the material with strong emotional charge and brings it into consciousness for processing'.[7] We've all experienced our physical body's innate capacity to heal itself and the Grofs find it no great stretch to believe this can happen for our psyche as well.

Lynsey provided a short orientation and introduced herself and her helpers. She asked us to choose a partner and spend a couple of minutes gazing silently into their eyes. I turned to Luke and gaze we did, an almost imperceptible grin passing over our faces from time to time, and I realised that Luke was the first person I've ever felt comfortable enough to engage in this surprisingly intimate act.

'The breathwork will go for 90 minutes, but don't worry, it'll feel quick,' Lynsey began introducing the main game. 'Just raise your hand if you need anything and one of us will be there for you. There'll be music playing throughout and I'll provide guidance at different points. I'll model the breathing techniques, as we go along. You're welcome to stop at any time if it feels too much for you.'

Before long, everyone in the room is breathing deeply in unison. Two minutes in, Lynsey makes her way over to me, winding her way through the yoga mats, and whispers in my ear:

'You're shaking a lot, is that normal for you?'

'Yes,' I nodded.

'Do you feel safe?' Lynsey checked.

'Very,' I replied.

My holotropic journey

I'm so conscious of Luke. I feel responsible. My spirit leaves my body to whoosh across and hug him tightly from underneath. I'm providing a safe container for him. This trip can be about him, not me—it's his first time.

But now, somehow reassured that Luke is okay, my spirit is released and flies over oceans, ravines, gorges, waterfalls, continents, taking in the beauty and wondrousness of the planet. I'm whizzing through scenes from my past, one after another, all random and without any particular pattern or meaning. My physical body keeps flinging itself upwards from the hip, in spontaneous sit-ups, and I feel my hands swell and tingle. The boundaries of my body dissolve and I turn into a dome of cushions that looks, in my mind's eye, like a giant tortoise. I'm so comfortable.

Now I'm back on the psilocybin retreat. I've landed back in the tripping room. It feels so vivid and real and great to be back with all those people and those euphoric feelings. And now I'm back on the Bufo retreat, tripping and loving the body sensations of billowing boundaries.

I start perceiving messages: it's all just fine exactly how it is. Three little words, 'let it be'. I repeat it ten, twenty times. I want to be this person. The person who can let it be and accept things as they are. My mind starts generating lists of recent irritations: doctor's waiting rooms, forms, banks, call centres, person X to deal with, person Y to deal with, others' moods and I understand it's possible to simply accept all the grievances with equanimity. I feel pure serenity and deep peace, happy to be in the moment, mind wandering nowhere.

At the end of the session several people shared their experiences with the group—breakthroughs, realisations, emotional releases, feelings of joy.

When it's over, Luke and I walk through the expanse of parkland adjoining the hall. The brief moment that I'd looked at Luke during the breathwork session, I'd seen his head had trembled slightly so I knew that something, and not 'nothing', had happened for him.

I opened the conversation: 'It's funny, comparing breathwork to taking a psychedelic. For me, it's a less intense experience. If someone had tapped me on the shoulder and told me I had to take an important phone call, I feel like I could've stood up at any point and snapped out of it. I wasn't deeply lost in it, even though it was amazing.'

Luke shared that, by the end, he felt a connection with everyone in the room.

He'd experienced several intense emotional states, revisited some painful times in his past, felt some body tremors. He was glad he'd done it. He was also exhausted for the rest of the day and would wake that night with random, unfamiliar pains in parts of his body that he felt sure related back to the workshop.

'Maybe you stirred up some old traumas,' I suggested.

'I know, the body keeps the score,' he echoed my constant refrain. 'I'm sure I did.'

I hoped he'd take further action on a psychedelic journey to continue processing whatever had started happening in his body, but I wouldn't pressure him. He had to feel the call.

Looking back, weeks down the track, I regarded my breathwork session as a series of treats—spectacular views, pleasant sensations, the insight to 'let it be'. It felt fun but, unlike many others in the room, I wouldn't be able to call it life-changing, or transformative or even particularly healing. Nor did I notice any changes in Luke, although who knows what mysterious blockages he may have released or stirred up. Holotropic breathers often have faith, or trust in the process, that even if they are unaware with the rational mind of what they gleaned from an experience, releases and shifts still occurred. As the Grofs write, 'The mind is the worst enemy', as breathers need to focus on 'emotions and physical sensations, refraining from intellectual analysis'.[8]

10

Lead-up to MDMA in Australia

It's not always easy, when I meet new people, to explain my current job exploring the world of psychedelics. You never know how they'll react. As I gradually meet Luke's friends, couple by couple, most have been open and curious. One mother of adult children sounded particularly accepting as she expressed a point I'd heard a few times, 'Oh yes, our son says, "Mum, if you go to a pub where everyone's drinking alcohol, there's often a hostile, aggressive vibe, but if you go somewhere where everyone's taking MDMA, everyone loves each other, they're affectionate and happy". It makes you wonder why alcohol is the legal one.'

Joe Rogan made a similar point in one of his podcasts:

> The one MDMA trip I had made me realise how insecure I was . . . I didn't realise how [my insecurities] affect every single interaction that I would have with people . . . There's this weird tension that human beings have when you first meet people but these people that I met when we were doing MDMA together, no-one had any fear. We were all holding hands and talking. It was this bizarrely free experience.[1]

I was surprised to hear Joe Rogan talk like this. If the most popular podcaster in the world, with his easy conversational style, his numerous friends and his career success—as a podcaster, comedian and fight commentator—had insecurities around his fellow human beings, how much more do the rest of us have?

MDMA has been shown to make even the most antisocial seek company—and by antisocial I mean the type capable of physically attacking their partner after sex. I write of the octopus, a creature that usually presents as an aggressive loner. An article entitled 'The undersea and the ecstasy', describes a study in which four octopuses absorbed MDMA from water through their gills.[2] Next, given a choice of three chambers, one empty, one with a toy and one with another octopus, all four swam to the cage with the other octopus, something they didn't do without MDMA in their system. Moreover, when on MDMA their movements were 'touchy-feely', 'relaxed and friendly' and 'playful' compared to 'tentative' without the MDMA.

How risky is MDMA?

Since July 2023, for those in Australia with a diagnosis of treatment-resistant post-traumatic stress syndrome (PTSD), MDMA has been legal as part of psychedelic-assisted psychotherapy, but this is extremely expensive. Otherwise, MDMA is only available through underground networks. The degree of contamination is way too high to justify the risk of taking it unless you have a pill-testing kit. The first Australian trial of pill-testing at a music festival occurred in 2018 at an event called Groovin the Moo. Of 85 pills submitted for testing, MDMA among many, only 50 per cent of them were pure and the tests identified two pills containing deadly substances along with paint and toothpaste.[3] The new drug-testing facility in Canberra, CanTEST, found in its first month that thirteen of nineteen samples of MDMA submitted for testing detected MDMA.[4] At the time of writing, the state of New South Wales is about to debate pill-testing at music festivals, while the states of Tasmania and Queensland have beaten them to it and allow it.

A research paper, 'MDMA-related deaths in Australia 2000 to 2018', informs us that over a period of eighteen years, 392 Australians died after taking MDMA:

> Two-thirds (62%) of deaths were attributed to drug toxicity (48% multiple drug toxicity and 14% MDMA toxicity alone), and one third (38%) to other causes (predominantly motor vehicle accidents) with MDMA recorded as a contributory factor. [5]

To be clear, 55 Australians died in that eighteen-year period from taking pure MDMA. I did some rough maths to ascertain the chance of dying from MDMA, taken with other drugs, to be 0.00004 per cent; and MDMA on its own to be 0.000008 per cent.[6] Driving my car, in Australia, puts my risk of death at 0.44 per cent.[7]

How interesting that as a culture we greatly emphasise drug risks and ignore some far higher risks in our daily activities. Neuropsychopharmacologist Professor David Nutt, for example, stated during a lecture in 2009 that both drinking alcohol and horse-riding were more dangerous than taking MDMA. He was immediately dismissed from his role on the Advisory Council on the Misuse of Drugs in the UK.[8]

Recreational users of MDMA dance (literally) with the possibly fatal dangers of overheating or overhydrating, not to mention the risk of inflicting lasting damage on their mental health and memory if they use it frequently enough to deplete their serotonin levels. That said, in all the legal, therapeutic settings there have been no fatalities, nor accidents, to date.[9]

Pioneering psychedelic researcher and psychiatrist Dr Rick Strassman (more about his work in chapter 19) wrote in *The Psychedelic Handbook* about recreational use of MDMA:

> Neurotoxicity [potential to cause brain damage] of MDMA is not a trivial issue . . . I treat the adverse effects of no other drug in this handbook in as much detail as I do with MDMA. The dividing line between the 'right amount' of MDMA and 'too much' is indistinct . . . It is probably safe to take pure MDMA in small to moderate doses a handful of times in one's life, perhaps even just once. However, regular, frequent, and heavy use is only asking for trouble.[10]

I decided that for myself, I'd try MDMA twice. Fate, however, would ultimately decide: for me, only once.

More about releasing

During my online search for an integration therapist to guide me through an MDMA trip, I chanced on a website called Psychedelic Passage for those in the United States who seek psychedelic guides. I needed an Australian version, but that didn't exist. The focus of the resources on the Psychedelic Passage site was squarely on the importance of set, setting, preparation, integration and all the usual safety considerations. I listened to a podcast by the founders of the site, Nick and Jimmy, which turned out to be the ideal preparation for the MDMA experience I was about to have. They credited the ideas they discussed to a book called *Waking the Tiger: Healing Trauma* by Peter Levine, a book I'd heard recommended several times including by the integration therapist I'd eventually settle with. Nick and Jimmy started their podcast conversation with the point that psychedelics help us 'release traumatic residue' from our bodies, particularly from our nervous systems.[11]

> **Nick:** . . . animals have these traumatic experiences all the time in nature, and they don't walk around with PTSD. So, what's the difference in humans? . . . animals listen to their instinctual need to discharge this excess energy from their nervous system and from their body. If you see an antelope after a cheetah chases it, the first thing it'll do, once it escapes, is lie down on

the ground, and oftentimes shake for an extended period of time before it gets back up and then goes out into the world.

We, as humans, typically don't allow ourselves to do this. I always joke with clients that if you, in the middle of your workday, started shaking and convulsing at your desk, that would probably cause alarm.

... What I see a lot of times with clients that I'm supporting during their journey is they have these very visceral somatic or bodily releases ... like trembling or shaking through the hands, feet, shoulders, chest, limbs, temperature fluctuations from hot to cold, excessive yawning, crying, spitting—

Jimmy: Mucus production, vocalisations ... mumbling, spontaneous movements in the body, feelings of tingling, feelings of almost like falling asleep, feeling a desire to get up and move, or desire to lay down and curl up in the fetal position, I do a ton of just rocking back and forth, and things like that. I like, can't sit still ... you're a yawner.

... Sometimes that's spontaneous crying. Some people are like, 'I'm crying, and I have no idea why but this feels so good.' And I'm like, 'Yes, keep going.' I'm cheering them on almost.

... You may not be able to define things like, 'Oh, this is my trauma from when I was five releasing.' You might not be able to put a finger on it, but there are different ways that we can discharge. I find that the heart space releasing is a common theme with the clients that I work with.

Another thing that I note is that in the female clients that I work with, regardless of whether it's trauma-informed work or not, there's often a lot of work in the throat space, I find that there's some commonality there.

My throat had always been the number one place for my spasming, which had started during meditation sessions, well before my psychedelic journey. A Buddhist teacher once told me that sensations in the throat area relate to self-expression. So, spasms in the throats of females, I've speculated, might relate to the way many women feel silenced, or unable to express themselves, due to their need to please others, never disappoint anyone and avoid conflict. Just saying.

Nick: Yeah. I've definitely experienced both of those with clients—the chest opening and the throat spasms. The most common stuff I see is involuntary muscle movements. But this to me is the act of your nervous system reregulating . . . [Psychedelics] . . . put us in this state of allowance. In other words, most of our defence mechanisms come from our default mode network, which is associated with this ego structure. And psychedelics reduce or turn off altogether that part of our brain . . . The nervous system goes, 'Oh, okay, all your defense mechanisms are offline, I'm finally going to get a chance to re-regulate in the way that I've been wanting to, but haven't had the space, the ability, the time or the permission to.

They discussed how we can fool our minds that we've resolved some inner crisis but our bodies know better.

Nick: [People I've worked with] . . . describe the feeling of being stuck. They're like, 'I know all these things, conceptually, mentally, but I can't seem to move past it or break the pattern or break the trigger, break the compulsion.

Jimmy: . . . you can fool your mind and you can change the narrative and the story around how you think about things and the emotions you feel around it. But you really can't fool the body . . . I actually saw this really funny meme that said, 'The Body Keeps the Score. Can someone tell the body that it's not a competition?'

Nick: We feel we must do something to address our past traumas but often we don't have to do anything. It's when we allow the body to discharge that things become unstuck . . . Talking is also not the only pathway [to deal with trauma], thinking is not the only pathway.

Jimmy: And it's important to say that it doesn't all happen in one psychedelic experience. If you've got a little internal traffic jam, meaning that you have not allowed yourself to discharge or express or feel or move in a way that you can naturally discharge this . . . if you are relying on peak experiences that have this discharge, but then in your normal life, you don't have any of that, well, it's all going to traffic jam again in your body.

I was reminded of the pain in my wrist, which had hurt so badly during my psilocybin trip and later in the final breathwork session of the Bufo retreat. The pain in the breathwork session was a way to continue the process of releasing, to continue clearing the traffic jam. Natasja had warned us that any psychoactive substances could re-activate aspects of our trip, and this happened whenever I took THC, the psychoactive part of cannabis, for my sleep. My mysterious wrist pain returned but each time the pain was a little less—as though the processing of the trauma was nearing completion, before it finally disappeared altogether. It was my body's 'inner healing intelligence' at work, to again quote Stan Grof of LSD and Holotropic Breathwork fame. I would probably never know what the wrist pain related to but apparently the not-knowing didn't matter.

As a side note, I question my right to talk about releasing trauma. Bessel van der Kolk, recognised expert on trauma (mentioned in chapter 2), took issue with the notion that every human could claim to be a victim of trauma. He felt the word should be reserved for victims of crime or abuse and those who'd suffered 'adverse childhood experiences'. I hadn't experienced such traumas, even if I'd had my share of misery, and I felt like a drama queen to speak of 'releasing my traumas'. Yet, it seemed to be standard in the psychedelic world to assume that trauma was part of the human condition, one's birth often being the first example.

The Buddha may have agreed that we all face trauma given his First Noble Truth was 'There is suffering'[12] and his examples of 'birth, sickness, aging and death'. Nick and Jimmy found a way around the conundrum by differentiating 'Big T trauma', in the case of experiences of abuse or violence from 'Little t trauma' for the accumulation of less life-threatening events.

Finding MDMA and an integration therapist

While there were no legal MDMA retreats in the world, I still wanted to take MDMA in an appropriate set and setting. I needed someone I could talk to for preparation and integration, who could provide the 'safe container' and guidance I'd appreciated on retreats. The only option available, given I was unlikely to qualify for any research trials, would be to find a professional guide. Plenty of psychologists, psychotherapists and counsellors in Australia offered 'psychedelic integration' on their websites as a service or, more often, one of several of their services. Their websites always included in capital letters that they DO NOT ENCOURAGE ANY ILLEGAL ACTIVITY NOR PROVIDE ANY ILLEGAL SUBSTANCES. Nor would most of them do any trip-sitting. Many of those I contacted for psychedelic integration had closed their books. Such is the demand for mental health services in the post-COVID world.

Eventually my search for an integration therapist bore fruit. Through word-of-mouth I chanced on Sasha and scheduled a phone call. I started with my usual spiel: 'I'm looking for someone who can provide preparation or integration sessions for some psychedelics I plan to take—I know you can't provide the psychedelic itself. I just wanted to find out about what you offer and whether you can do the therapy on Zoom, for example.'

'Sure, I'm a psychotherapist by training and I've been doing psychedelic integration work for the last two or three years,' Sasha introduced herself.

'How did you get into it?' I asked.

'I know the power of psychedelics personally and I found them to be a gateway into parts of the self that are hard to access. I gradually started working with friends and would go on to hold space for people at music festivals. In my psychotherapy work I've found the medicines allow clients to get into new relationships with different parts of themselves.'

'So, what do your therapy sessions look like?'

'I do inner child work, I work holistically and try to work deeply with my clients—I also provide psilocybin and MDMA if a patient wants them as those medicines have the greatest potential for transformation.'

Had I heard her properly?

'I'm interested,' I replied, moving to the edge of my seat. 'I've struggled to find a safe source of MDMA so it'd be amazing if I could feel assured of its safety. I bought it through informal contacts not long ago but it didn't pass my pill-testing kit.'

'Yes, we take safety very seriously and only use reputable, clean sources,' Sasha stated in a steady voice that I couldn't help but trust. I wondered who 'we' was only to discover her partner was also a qualified psychotherapist, and underground guide, and one whose background I was quite familiar with through my research. They'd even run underground Bufo retreats together. I inquired about her availability.

'I'm quite heavily booked for the coming weeks and I won't be around after August as I'll be having a baby. Standard practice for me is three preparation sessions beforehand and three integration sessions afterwards.'

I had to act fast. I made some tectonic changes to my schedule to make it happen. Sasha lived far away so we scheduled my first Zoom preparation session. I'd need to travel interstate but looked forward to escaping the Sydney winter for warmer climes.

Me and therapy

I knew that engaging in therapy was the safest and most responsible way to take this illegal substance. If the police arrested me, and I stood in court for the crime of trying to do some work on my own mind, I could say that I was pursuing 'harm minimisation' by modelling how to take a substance safely. Australian drug policy, after all, has been one of 'harm minimisation' since 1985.[13]

The thing is: I hate therapy.

I fear I'm more work than any counsellor can handle. In the darkest moments of my life, I've reached out to psychologists only to quit after a couple of sessions. In my last job everyone in my role was required to see a therapist, or 'supervisor', once a month. I tried a couple but, again, quit soon after starting.

I felt like my underlying problems, my various self-doubts and insecurities, were too entrenched to ever go away so what would be the point of focusing on them, which only felt like going round in never-ending circles without getting anywhere. Through my Buddhist practice, my study of psychology, and conversations with the wise, I believed I'd developed enough self-awareness to manage my demons, to ensure they rarely harmed others. I was confident that I loved, liked and (usually) respected myself. That said, I still feel like a ding-a-ling most of the time.

I saw MDMA, and the therapy and self-focus that would accompany it, as a pitstop before ayahuasca, to do a bit more cleaning out of my system. After all, MDMA was not technically a member of the class of drugs called 'psychedelics', but rather an 'empathogen', a term that emphasises its capacity to generate empathy, for one's self and others. Dr Strassman in *The Psychedelic Handbook* had said the effects of MDMA 'differ from the classical compounds in that perceptual alterations and disruption of the normal sense of self are significantly less pronounced with MDMA than are its emotional properties'.

I wasn't expecting a big experience with MDMA and had planned a long bus trip home the next day followed by a week of appointments and commitments.

How wrong I turned out to be.

Therapy with Sasha

I sat at my desk five minutes early for the Zoom with my new psychotherapist Sasha. I had the usual mild anxiety that arises when I meet someone for the first time and don't know what to expect. I only know that I'll need to reveal parts of myself that are usually hidden and this might make me feel overexposed and vulnerable.

Suddenly a face appeared in front of me.

'Hi Sasha!' I opened, hopefully looking cool and breezy.

The first thing I thought is how lucky she is. So healthy and natural, she has no need for all the makeup I've plastered on my face; and those intellectual glasses give her a gravitas inviting instant respect.

After some niceties I decided to be honest.

'I'm actually the happiest I've ever been. All my old wounds were much more of an issue in the past. I know they're still there but it's tempting to skip all the trouble of reviving them and opt for repression instead. I feel like I could easily get away with that.'

'Yes, doing the work, it's not fun,' Sasha replied. 'It feels messy and it's normal to want to stop and quit, at times. Can I ask, how do you think repression would feel for you, at this stage in your life?'

'Well, I'm 55 years old. These issues have been around my whole life. If I haven't sorted them out by now, can it ever happen?'

'I've had clients in their sixties and seventies . . .'

It was a good question. How would repression feel? It was extremely rare these days that I 'dropped my bundle' or had a 'meltdown', but even so it could happen. Usually triggered by a combination of sleep-deprivation and some form of interpersonal conflict, I'm capable of ugly-crying and levels of self-pity that embarrass me to reflect back on. Moreover, I still wanted to feel more connected to my fellow human beings, but something mysterious (sometimes not so mysterious) prevented me. Maybe I should embrace this therapy process more. We agreed we would work on deciding on an intention for the MDMA trip.

'Well,' I began, 'I had a look, an hour or two ago, at this list of 28 things I'd change about myself that I wrote a few months ago and I used a highlighter to find some common themes. I found ten of them related to interpersonal or relationship problems, five of them related to feelings of inadequacy and thirteen of them related to things like stress/rush/impatience/overwhelm—that kind of thing. I guess they're all themes you're familiar with in your work?'

Sasha nodded slowly and emphatically, as a knowing grin warmed her face.

'Definitely,' she replied, 'and we often find that themes like that are interrelated. Fixing one can do a lot for the others as well.'

'That's interesting. Can you give an example?' I asked.

'Well, people may feel the need to rush, and be constantly stressed, only because their early parental relationships left them feeling they weren't good enough to meet their parents' expectations. So, the stressing and the interpersonal difficulty overlap.'

While that precise scenario didn't apply to me, I understood her point.

'So, of those three themes you identified,' Sasha asked, 'is there one you've noticed coming up for you lately? That you find yourself dwelling on?'

'I'm probably still processing some interpersonal issues. My intentions for the Bufo ceremony a couple of months ago had been about coping with some social rejection. While there were some breakthroughs from the Bufo, I still feel some residual pain regarding one final friend I'm struggling to let go of. Her name's Rebecca.'

'Yes, I can hear the pain in your voice. Where do you feel that in your body right now?'

'Definitely in the chest, the heart area.'

'Good. We often go into our head to avoid the trauma stored in our body but that leaves the suffering trapped in our bodies unaddressed. We need to keep landing back in the body.'

I was starting to feel a tad choked up and vulnerable. I told Sasha more about feeling, in days gone by, that there was nobody there for me when I felt my worst and about how I would often feel painfully disconnected from the human race. Some part of me felt overwhelmed, however, and I shifted the conversation to lighter matters.

'I like that phrase: to land in the body,' I reflected.

'Yes, it's important to stay connected to the body and check in with it throughout the day. A lot of us find the brain a place of safety and use it to avoid what's happening in our bodies. It helps to ask at various points throughout the day, what am I feeling in my body? We need to keep energy moving through our body and notice what subtle movements we need to make in any given moment—perhaps a stretch, a shrug, a twist.'

The body, again. It had been a recurring theme on my psychedelic journey and I had to admit I needed these constant reminders. It would take many of them to stop my habit of trying to think, or talk, my way out of problems. Maybe past therapy had failed for me because it stayed at the head level and neglected the body—where it was all happening.

'Whenever you feel yourself getting overwhelmed,' Sasha continued, 'land back in your body. I tell clients to stamp their feet on the floor, in a kind of marching motion, as a way to feel their body again or as a way to ground themselves in the present. It's also really effective to cross your arms as if to give yourself a tight, firm hug. Your body calms down in response to a hug whether it comes from yourself or another. Some people benefit from using a weighted blanket to feel grounded and less flighty.'

'I have to say, my body is always restless, and achy, unless I get loads of exercise every single day; and if you asked me at any point in the day what I want more than anything in the world the answer is always: a good massage.'

'Sounds like you have lots of stored energy in there,' Sasha observed.

'So, what does MDMA add to the healing process?' I asked.

'It helps you feel the things you usually avoid feeling. It allows you to integrate all your parts including the wounded parts. It lets you access parts of yourself that can be hard to reach. At one point in my life, for example, I used to enjoy taking MDMA and going out dancing, but every time, I'd have to leave the dance area and engage with some profound experience that arose within me. You can meet these vulnerable parts of yourself and allow the grown-up part to enter into a relationship with it.'

'It almost sounds like you're dividing yourself into two. Like there's this maternal part that's going to look after its child.'

'That's exactly it. We often speak of re-parenting.'

In Buddhism there was frequent talk of *multiple* selves (if any self at all) as opposed to the one monolithic self we routinely assume runs the show. Multiple personality disorder also came to mind. There had been a heroic trauma victim in the courts where I worked who had made headlines all over the world when each of her different personalities was granted permission to give evidence in their different voices. She appeared on the stand as five-year-old Symphony and then later as teenage boy Muscles. I digress.

'One really important thing,' Sasha continued, 'is to make sure there's a way to nurture the grown-up part too after your trip. It's good to have some supports lined up. Do you feel you have some resources?'

'Yeah, no problem there. I talk a lot to my partner about these things and I meditate, spend time in nature, do breathwork, mindfulness of the body, yoga . . .'

I stopped after one preparation session instead of Sasha's usual three. I was still determined to avoid therapy. I would later, however, need more than one integration session.

11

MDMA in Queensland

A WEEK AFTER MY Zoom therapy with Sasha, I treated myself to a day or two wandering along the palm-fringed beaches of Queensland, but the weather was grey—as was my mood. The beauty of nature failed to move me—the lookouts, the forest trails, even the occasional distant dolphins, were all lost on me, although three sea turtles bobbing around the shoreline distracted me for a few moments.

Luke and I had been together almost two years, most of that time living together, but now cracks had appeared. To protect my precious mindset, I'd blocked him on my phone, which I knew he wouldn't appreciate, but it was too late: my mindset was ruined. I felt anxious as I catastrophised that the relationship might be over and I'd be completely alone. I struggled to picture a future devoid of the laughter, fun and intimacy we'd enjoyed.

MDMA trip

Sasha entered my tiny, rented studio unit, which was dominated by a king-size bed complete with white cushions and a puffy white doona. We took a kitchen chair each to prepare for the trip ahead. I bombarded her with questions to which she tended to answer, 'Whatever feels right for you.'

'I've been reading the book you recommended, *Waking the Tiger*,' I told Sasha. 'It seems to be about Big T trauma where someone has survived a traumatic incident, or abuse, but I don't feel that applies to me. There have been difficulties in my life, and my fair share of loneliness, but others have suffered more than me.'

'Thinking back on our last conversation, though,' Sasha began, 'to lack a sense of belonging, to not get your emotional needs met, is deeply, deeply painful. That's a kind of trauma.'

To hear the words 'deeply, deeply painful' struck a chord for me. I agreed, disconnection from those around you can be deeply, deeply painful. Then I confessed.

'I'm afraid I haven't come into this with the best mindset. I've been feeling triggered by a few things in the last few days. Thoughts of that friend who dumped me, Rebecca, and—'

'Yes, before a trip it's as though our nervous system knows, on some level, that something big is about to happen,' Sasha observed.

'My mindset's pretty bad, to tell you the truth. I've been having some relationship tension with Luke and it's made my mood very, um, flat.'

'I know what you mean. My partner and I trigger the shit out of each other.'

I loved her for that line; for too many reasons to list. Not least, it helped me to feel understood.

'You never know,' Sasha offered, 'sometimes it's what's supposed to happen. You'll still have the journey you need. Have you thought about your intention?'

'I've found it hard to come up with something concise but I guess it'd be something like: to address the loneliness from my past, or to ease my dread of loneliness in the future or something like that.'

Preparation complete, we stood up and Sasha handed me a clear capsule with a few black flakes inside, 100 micrograms. I swallowed it down with water, adjusted the volume on the headphones, put my eye mask on, and slid under the doona.

Well, it's taking a while to come on, it feels like twenty minutes, at least. She's chosen super-slow, floaty music. I do like the way I'm seeing the notes as colourful swirls. These visuals are bejewelled and beautiful but they are under the cover of darkness—I haven't seen this black theme before. Gee, I can't believe how comfortable my body feels—it's so pleasant to feel cocooned in softness at every contour. It feels like being held, in kindness, gentleness and love. I'm so loved and cherished. Thank you, Thank you, Thank you—I repeat dozens of times over. I feel so much gratitude to be one of the few allowed to feel these feelings. So cared for. My eyes tear up. This is a bliss I've never felt before.

I hear moans. Like a baby crying. The moans emanate from me, but I don't feel the baby's sadness. I listen to the moans escaping my mouth and want so badly to comfort the sad baby. I channel my feelings of bliss and love into the moaning infant for what feels like a very long time. I stroke the baby. I cuddle the baby. I hold her close. The baby is me, of course. As I listen to the moans, I realise they are the moans I made in my first psilocybin trip, when I'd blacked out, and everyone heard them except me. How fascinating to hear what everyone in that psilocybin-trip room had heard. I recall their compassion—and my amazement at their compassion.

Now I'm the toddler in her bed who is done screaming and realises that nobody will come and comfort her. My adult self snuggles up to her, holds her close and whispers reassurance. Adult Sarah promises to look after the toddler from now on. I return to the moaning baby and walk her around a room, bouncing her up and down, whispering words of love in her ear.

Comforting the baby, comforting the toddler, I feel bliss and continue to channel the immense love into the youngsters. My moans turn from sounds of distress to sounds of comfort, cooing, mewling.

Now that the little ones are at peace, I go back and visit various painful scenes from my life, a series of snapshots. Yet none of these scenes mar the bliss, gratitude and wonder. I'm strong enough to go anywhere. Nowhere is too painful. Everything will be okay. Unassailable love prevails.

Now Rebecca's face appears, my lost friend. She smiles and looks twenty years younger, radiant. I smile into her face and say, 'Goodbye Rebecca' and she says, 'Bye Sarah' smiling back at me. We hug and I know I'm over her now. We've said our final goodbye. It felt good, it felt right. I replay the scene, for good measure and feel an exhilarating release. I wish her well and know she does the same for me.

I see the face of my oldest friend, Viv, and cry my gratitude to her for standing by me, through all my idiocies, since primary school. I utter a dozen thank yous.

I see Marek and embrace him, full of platonic love.

I see Luke and hear the message, 'This one's not going to last'.

Where did that come from? I ask, surprised. It felt clear, unambiguous. Still, I see images of his face and feel compassion.

For the first time in the trip, I speak to my guide Sasha, 'Do you have Spotify?'

'I do'.

'I don't usually like Coldplay but could you play . . . I think it's called 'Lights Will Guide You Home', or 'Kiss You', or 'Kick You' or something.'

Seconds later . . .

'"Fix You"?' Sasha asks.

'Yes, thank you.'

Every time the song ends, I ask her to play it again. Eight times, in all. Whenever the song reaches its crescendo my body shudders violently and as it slows down for the final line, I burst into tears. All eight times.

The final line of the song is a slow 'I will try to fix you'. The first few times I understand it as the voice of the Divine talking to me. By around the fifth listen I realise it's the Divine inside me talking to Baby Sarah, Toddler Sarah and Grown-Up Sarah: 'I will try to fix you.' I realise I've been a broken person. Far more broken than I've admitted in a long time. You poor, poor thing, I mutter. But looking after all the parts of myself, from this point on, I may well be fixed.

That night I slept badly, as I knew I would. I'd spent the daylight hours lying in bed, after all, so my body had no need for sleep.

Thoughts swirled: *How can governments not want us to feel those feelings? I need to spread the word, yell from the mountaintops. I need to administer MDMA to my loved ones. Heck, I could end up in gaol but if I could help any suffering people to access those feelings, I'd be honoured to go to gaol! Oh dear, I'll need to find a way to curb my enthusiasm.*

I made a mental list of all the people I wanted to give MDMA to. With so much grind and struggle in even the best of lives, why can't people have some of this for relief? I reflected on the bliss; I'd never experienced that emotion: unconditional happiness, a happiness independent of any who, what, why or where. Nothing needed. Nothing to add. Perfect, perfect happiness. How could such an experience not help the sad and lonely out there? I'd been pretty depressed myself right before the trip and look how that changed.

I rose from bed at 5 a.m. and, on autopilot, threw back two strong coffees, my customary gift to myself after a bad night's sleep, as I usually drink tea.

To my surprise, I'm not done tripping, and my body goes on a journey of its own, independent of my mind. I pace the room, hug myself standing up, hug myself lying down, cradle my violently shuddering torso, notice my head wobbles and, of course, grind my teeth. What's different about this MDMA trip, however, is the involuntary vocalisations. I make a cacophony of sounds. I have no idea what sound will spill out next, but spill they do. Baby Sarah whimpering, dramatic inhales, noisy exhales, shuddering groans, raspberries, whooshes of breath, puffing, strange made-up words: tica-tica-tica-tica, ca-ca-ca-ca, yelps, gulps.

Eventually I decide to have a shower and something sweet happens. I sing aloud, but it's not the kind of song any adult would sing. It's one of those tunes that children make up as they go along, the kind you hear a four-year-old sing as they play with their Lego—in no particular key, with no particular melody. My adult mind tries to impose sensible notes but the singing child won't accept them—she knows what she wants to sing and no grown-up is going to get in her way. She's such a happy little girl.

The singing eventually ends. I stand and hug myself but burst into tears, grown-up tears. I'm suddenly overwhelmed. I also have a bus to catch soon but I can't stop shuddering and moaning. I pack and make my way to the bus stop, which is fortunately close by, and in the middle of nowhere, so I can wait for the bus in privacy. I feel horrible—a little scared that my mind is unhinged and I shouldn't be out and about. I wish I knew what was going on with me. I wait half an hour alone hoping that my spasming body and all the involuntary moaning will settle down by the time the bus arrives.

Who makes these moaning sounds from my mouth? I wonder. Is it grown-up Sarah? One of the sexual assault victims from my old job? An ancestor, or a character from one of my past lives? I'm stumped. Suddenly, I realise that I probably shouldn't have had two coffees. I google 'MDMA and coffee' and see enough website titles to know I've done something really stupid. I've committed something called 'polydrug use'—taken a mixture of drugs, and this is really unsafe. I wonder if I've undone all the good work of yesterday's trip.

When the bus arrives it's half full and I beeline for the back. The bus has a noisy engine, which protects the public from my noises and I'm alone at the back. A few stops later a bunch of noisy skateboarders join me on the back seat but they don't seem to notice me or hear me, too busy teasing each other and playing music on their phones. This doesn't stop one of them from somehow leaving an enormous wad of chewing gum on my luggage, which I'd discover later strung across my thighs.

For the whole bus trip home my mood is terrible and I'm cross with myself about those coffees. I'd heard that the 'comedown' from MDMA could be harsh but now I would never know if my terrible mood, and the ongoing moaning, was part of the comedown or simply due to my 'polydrug use', or both.

I arrived home late at night and fell into bed only to wake at around 2 a.m. The final few bars of Mike Oldfield's *Tubular Bells,* with its heavenly choirs, entered my mind and I'm back on a happy trip, comforting the baby, hugging the toddler, enjoying the bliss and the comforting body sensations. The next day too, I know I'm still under the influence and enjoy another two pleasantly trippy interludes. And the day after that as well.

Integration Zoom with Sasha

Four days after the MDMA trip, Sasha appears on my screen. She's so telegenic.

'I have so much to talk about, Sasha. A lot's happened, but I think I need to vent first. The tension with Luke has continued.'

I'll spare you, reader, the 'he-said-she-said' details and fast-forward to: 'I finally told him what had been getting at me before I left for Queensland and then I announced I was going to take a walk in the park to allow him time to process what I'd said. So, I was walking around the park but I was amazed that I felt light and happy. Usually, at moments like that, mid-conflict, I fall into a deep well of despair, anxiety and depression. Whenever there's conflict, I suffer from that condition *can't-stand-it-itis.* Not this time. I felt breezy. I smiled as I walked round the park and I knew my lightness was because the baby inside had been comforted and wasn't scared of abandonment anymore. The vulnerable baby, and toddler, inside had been comforted.'

Sasha smiled broadly and I knew she was happy for me. 'How did you feel straight after you told Luke you were going to the park to give him time?'

'I felt a huge expansiveness instead of the usual rising panic.'

I told Sasha about how, despite my upbeat mood, the tension with Luke hadn't been resolved yet and I wasn't sure what to do—I couldn't see a way out of our issues.

'It's normal,' Sasha responded, 'to gravitate to people who trigger us. I think the important question is, can we still grow together? Can we do the work together? Take responsibility? Does a partner allow you the space to grow? There can be growth in staying together, but also in leaving. Or even leaving for a while to create some space. Of course, you need to feel safe and appreciated—'

I could vouch that there were no safety issues with Luke and until recently we'd both felt deeply appreciated by each other.

I told Sasha about the two cups of coffee, the morning after my trip, and how, after that, I kept falling back into a trip, twice a day or in the middle of the night. The moaning noise had only stopped today, four days later.

'How did you feel about continuing to trip like that?' Sasha asked.

'Some of the trips were blissful,' I replied, 'but a couple of them were annoying especially the shuddering and moaning. I couldn't believe how many sounds I was making—it was like Tourette's syndrome. I never knew what was going to come out next.'

'Clearly, something's opened up in you,' Sasha explained. 'Something's wanted to be expressed—a part of you that's been locked away. It's important to have a voice and it sounds like you've found it.'

'I have to say though that it was such a relief,' I told her, 'to wake up to no more moaning today. It was strange, though, that the symptoms—like all the noises and shaking—disappeared during my physio appointment yesterday, and last night when I had to lead a group meditation and discussion. I'd been so worried I'd act weirdly in front of others but somehow the symptoms knew to stop. What's a standard comedown from MDMA? Is it normal to keep tripping like this?'

'No, it's not normal. I'd say it was probably the effects of the coffee, which is a stimulant, and possibly the lack of sleep mixed in as well. Usually, in a therapeutic setting, the comedown is not particularly intense. You may just feel low energy or a flat mood from the decrease in serotonin. A harsh comedown is more likely when you've taken MDMA at a party. In that case you may not have slept, you may have danced and become dehydrated or, included alcohol in the mix.'

'Gee, I'm a bit of a special case then.'

'It seems like something was wanting to come through. Focus now on grounding yourself. Anchor yourself in your body, stomp your feet, hug yourself, hydrate. MDMA will heighten your nervous system, so you need to nourish yourself well with good foods, like broths, soups and healthy home cooking.'

I didn't admit I'd had the munchies and eaten lots of chips.

'In less than three weeks,' I blurted, 'Luke and I are leaving for Costa Rica to travel for three weeks together. I don't know what to do.'

We talked some more and, given my quandary with Luke, I was keen to schedule more therapy for the following week.

Big decisions

As with the advice at the end of Buddhist retreats, the advice after taking psychedelics is to avoid making any big decisions. With MDMA I was breaking all the rules: I had a bad mindset before the trip; I had underestimated the intensity of the experience and scheduled a long bus trip and other diary items for the following week, and next I would make a whopping great decision.

As the tension with Luke continued, and our differences proved irreconcilable, we agreed there was no choice but to break up. This meant I would also need to move out and find a new home somewhere. So much for not making any big decisions, Sarah. I'd also need to take that fully booked three-week holiday with Luke before

I moved out. I'd suggested during our final arguments that we travel in Costa Rica as friends and do our best to make it work, an approach he agreed to.

A couple of weeks before taking MDMA, there'd been a hint that a breakup was imminent and I'd cried like a baby for one or two hours. Now, just under a week after taking MDMA, the breakup had happened yet I felt calm, emotionally untouchable. I looked forward to the freedom and fresh start ahead, not least, the chance to reunite with some neglected hobbies. What had changed in me? Was it that the vulnerable baby inside, who feared abandonment, was finally at peace? Or was it that my amygdala, the fear centre of the brain, was still on extended leave? Was it that the default mode network had gone quiet and reduced the sense of any 'self' to be hurt? All three? I was so amazed at how peaceful I felt as I went about my day.

Lying in bed at four one morning, I had to admit that there would be many lonely hours ahead, many empty weekends to fill, but that would be a problem for Future Sarah. In these early hours, I didn't feel 100 per cent certain that this breakup would stick—would I weaken while in Costa Rica as we watched a sunset from a hammock on the beach? Still, I felt 80 per cent certain the breakup was final. When I meditated, I still tried to cultivate compassion for Luke and didn't find it hard.

In my next integration Zoom I told Sasha about the breakup and how, to my surprise, I felt fabulous: 'It's as though the breakup happened years ago—I'm simply not feeling very emotionally affected. I compare that to the emotional wreck I was a few weeks ago at the slightest hint of a breakup. Does that mean it will suddenly hit me one day when the MDMA wears off?'

'Not necessarily,' Sasha answered. 'You have new imprints in your mind now to replace the old imprints which triggered sadness and pain.'

'I do know there will be times of loneliness ahead—a few too many long Sundays alone, for example, or wanting to share some news, or some feelings, but having nobody there to tell.'

'The lonely feeling is really normal,' Sasha offered. 'Feeling sad and alone is part of being human. We can validate it whenever it comes up. Parent yourself. Be present, and attentive, to the feelings.'

'Even though I've always practised self-compassion as part of my meditation practice, I feel like my self-compassion is so much deeper now. I had no idea how deep it could go and how strong it could feel. I just imagine myself comforting that baby, that toddler and even my present-day self—it's a blissful feeling I can access whenever I feel like it.'

'Yes.' Sasha smiled. 'That often happens with the medicines. You assume you've mastered some spiritual or psychological teaching, only to find yourself going so much deeper than you ever thought possible.'

Psilocybin and MDMA had taught me that when we leave a baby to cry, there may be scars. While I couldn't remember any specific instances of leaving Alex to cry, I had a sneaky suspicion that, on occasion, I probably had. As a baby and a toddler, he'd cried so much and I'm sure there would've been times when I gave up and left him to it. Now, of course, I felt the guilt.

'I'm worried that maybe I harmed you in some way,' I admitted one day to Alex after explaining my trips to him.

'I guess we'll never know.' Alex shrugged. He didn't seem too perturbed, but now I'll always wonder.

The body

As the week after MDMA progressed, I marvelled at how light and supple my body felt. All those involuntary movements—the shuddering, clenching, spasming, not to mention all the sounds I'd made—had allowed my body to release stored tension. I now felt the benefit: I was no longer achy, restless Sarah. Physically and psychologically, I was a new person. Even the breakup couldn't diminish my feelings of renewal.

The sciatica in my right leg had gone. It had disappeared for three weeks after Bufo only to return. This time it disappeared for good. Whatever 'trauma' had been stored there was now fully processed.

MDMA for couples

It had been a long-running dream of mine to take MDMA with Luke. It was common knowledge what a beautiful, restorative experience taking MDMA could be for couples but now we'd broken up.

The best endorsement for MDMA as a love drug comes from Ayelet Waldman whose book *A Really Good Day* is a diary about her experiences microdosing LSD to treat a mood disorder despite her initial fear of illicit drugs. My favourite chapter was the one about MDMA where Waldman states, 'We credit the strength of our marriage at least in part to our periodic use of the drug'.[1] If you want a sense of 'the strength of our marriage', I can tell you that she was once a pariah among parents the world over for saying she loved her husband more than her children. She'd written the article 'Truly, Madly, Guiltily' for *The New York Times* in 2005 but I remember reading it in *The Sydney Morning Herald*.[2] She'd also claimed in the article that she could survive the death of a child, but not that of her husband.

Waldman describes an MDMA experience with her husband as six hours of talking about how much they love each other—an experience they revisit every couple of years. She concluded, regarding their first time with MDMA: 'The feeling lasted not for hours or for days, but for months. Actually, the truth is, it lasted forever.'

As well as being a mother of four, Waldman was a legal expert who at one point ran a university seminar on the war on drugs. One day, she invited pharmacologist Alexander Shulgin, the 'Father of MDMA' and the chemist credited with popularising the substance, to speak to her students. He spoke of how he shared the drug with a psychotherapist friend, Leo Zeff, who would train 'hundreds, perhaps even thousands, of therapists' to administer the substance in a therapeutic context. Shulgin spoke at the seminar along with his wife Ann who was experienced in providing MDMA in her couples counselling practice. Ann told the students she could 'accomplish more in a single six-hour session with MDMA than in six years of traditional therapy'. In 1985, MDMA in the United States was banned for recreational and therapeutic use, and the world would follow their lead.

Perhaps the most striking benefit that MDMA can offer couples is the chance to discuss hot topics without the usual defensiveness, anger and general reactivity.

It raised the question, what if you took MDMA with the wrong person only to have an unideal relationship strengthened? I don't know the answer, but I know that in my own trip, although I'd felt compassion for Luke as a fellow human, I'd received a clear message: this one's not going to last.

In the meantime, we were off to Costa Rica.

God help us.

12

Lead-up to ayahuasca in Costa Rica

It's amazing enough that there are plants that contain molecules that fit perfectly with receptors in our brains to provide the possibility of a mystical, mind-revealing or life-transforming experience. Ayahuasca is doubly amazing in that it's a combination of two plants working together, and from all the myriad plants in the Amazonian rainforest, the indigenous people managed to put the right two together. Of course, they believe they received divine assistance and it's hard to imagine they didn't.

In an ayahuasca ceremony I'd drink a tea made from the leaves of the *Psychotria viridis* plant, which contains the psychedelic DMT (dimethyltryptamine) and has a similar structure to the neurotransmitter serotonin. An enzyme in our saliva (monoamine oxidase) instantly breaks down the DMT to make it inactive, but if we add the boiled bark of the vine *Banisteriopsis caapi* it stops that enzyme breaking down the DMT.[1] This allows for an approximately six-hour communion with Mama Ayahuasca.

In the Native Indian language of Quechua, the 'aya' in ayahuasca means 'souls' or 'dead' or 'spirits,' while 'huasca' means 'vine'. So we can translate ayahuasca as 'vine of the dead', 'vine of the souls' or 'vine of the spirits'.[2] YouTube videos can help with pronunciation, or try: eye-ya-wuss (rhymes with bus)-car (with a silent 'r').

The usual country for drinking ayahuasca is Peru, in the depths of the Amazonian jungle in one of the hundreds of indigenous communities. In 2023, however, that country was in a state of political crisis with no end of violent protests, fatalities and roadblocks. Luke, my newly 'ex'-boyfriend, had decided months ago to use his annual leave to accompany me to South America, and given it'd be winter in Sydney, somewhere warm, north of the equator made sense. The tiny Central American country of Costa Rica offered plenty of ayahuasca retreats so Luke would travel with me for three weeks and then return home, leaving me to travel alone for a couple more weeks and attend the one-week retreat.

With a population just over 5 million, Costa Rica is two-thirds the size of Tasmania. The small land area would not rule out a busy holiday given its 30 national parks, six active volcanoes, 30 dormant ones, and the abundance of wildlife including sloths and giant turtles that you can watch at night laying hundreds of eggs. The Caribbean Sea lies along its east coast and the Pacific Ocean along the West, so there would be a choice of over 200 beaches.

Luke and I would need to educate ourselves about Costa Rica. Throughout my marriage, Marek had always consumed two and a half hours a day of world news and current affairs, a lot of which he shared with me at mealtimes, but I only remembered Costa Rica coming up once. They'd won the happiest country in the world award. In fact, they'd won that award four times. The Happy Planet Index website enthuses:

> Strong social networks, investment in health and education, and a deep connection to nature may help explain why Costa Ricans are happier and live longer than the residents of most wealthy nations. A national commitment to environmental protection and use of renewable energy also keeps Costa Rica's Ecological Footprint small.[3]

My guidebook indicated they'd reached almost 100 per cent renewable energy, through using mainly hydro power. They'd abolished their army back in 1948, freeing up funds to invest in the environment and education.[4] The paradise has its dark side, however, as for over a decade, drug gangs from South America have used Costa Rica as a waystation for cocaine and methamphetamine trafficking on their way to the United States.[5]

Since the year 2010, possessing drugs for personal use in Costa Rica has not been a criminal offence.[6] As for ayahuasca, the law is unclear, and no amount of googling could clarify it for me. DMT, which is a component of ayahuasca, is on the list of prohibited substances but there had been no sign of any legal threats to the dozens of ayahuasca retreat centres operating freely there.

Choosing a retreat

Months before our journey, I'd googled for hours to select a retreat, prioritising 'reasonable cost' and 'workable dates for Luke's work', while Luke repeated the mantra, 'safety first', often adding, 'it doesn't matter if the retreat costs hundreds more if it prioritises your safety'. Three people I respected from the Bufo retreat had suggested a retreat called Soltara but that was booked out. I grew frustrated until I read an article written by an American mother who ran a website from Costa Rica specialising in travel information for visiting families. An article on ayahuasca retreats was slightly outside her usual focus but she wrote:

> If you are a woman traveling alone or with a group of women, you will want to make sure there is a woman on staff to guide you through your journey. Both Nada Brahma Healing Center and Casa de la Luz specialize in creating a safe environment for women on site . . . The times I have spent at ayahuasca retreats have given me a strong peace of mind and relaxation. (I've never tried ayahuasca but have spent time at Nada Brahma Healing Center) . . . I have to say that I am completely biased about this retreat, but the shaman, Carlos, has been a family friend for over 20 years. His level of knowledge and professionalism is unparalleled, and his prices are the best on this list. If you are looking for a high-quality, authentic and intimate experience, stop reading now and just book with Carlos. Tell him Christa sent you![7]

This felt like a word-of-mouth recommendation, from a woman who'd known the shaman personally for two decades. I couldn't help but trust Christa who'd won me over with a mix of girl-next-door charm smiling from her website's photo plus her mention of safety and price, which both appeased Luke and appealed to me.

Some of the retreats I'd looked at offered six ayahuasca ceremonies but I knew that would be more vomiting than my sensitive person could handle. At Nada Brahma, there'd be three, which seemed more moderate. Numbers were limited to eight or nine retreatants, which suggested they were committed to quality care. Other retreats in Costa Rica took 80 people so you could only hope they had a good ratio of facilitators to retreatants. I watched videos of Carlos talking to a camera on YouTube and found his outlook chimed with Buddhism and its focus on the absence of a 'self' that we all assume is running our lives. A little cheaper than Natasja's retreats, there would be fewer 'extras', such as group Zooms before and after, but all testimonials on YouTube emphasised the high level of care and support.

As with Natasja's retreats, there'd be a preparation diet 'to allow the plant medicine to work more easily in your body'. It looked even more strict than the psilocybin diet. In the week leading up to the retreat I'd need to refrain from: all meat, caffeine, dairy, fried/processed/canned/fermented food and sweets, salt, vitamins, supplements and medications. Oh, and no sex in that week either. Note to self, book accommodation for the week before with a kitchen for a diet of boiled eggs, nuts, fruit and steamed vegetables. Bless the abundant avocados which would, at least, allow for some tasty guacamole.

I'd need to share a room, which seemed the norm on retreats everywhere. We could bring a notebook for journalling, but electronic devices and even books were not allowed. As usual, the medical form screened out people with diagnoses of schizophrenia, bipolar or any history of psychosis for whom the effects of the medicines were not yet fully researched. Some interesting inclusions were nutritional consultations, *unlimited time* with staff for integration after each ceremony and a complimentary laundry service.

There'd be no retreat schedule. As the introductory email said:

> We will begin to let you know what activities and medicine will be done as we go and as we feel the energy from the guests. You will let go of the concept of time.

Travelling in Costa Rica

Travelling as a recently broken-up couple proved intolerable. I felt crushed by feelings of guilt: this was Luke's precious annual leave; he'd so looked forward to a holiday for which he'd booked most of our accommodation and activities; he'd spent a small fortune, as had I, to come here. Yet neither of us could relax in each other's company and on a couple of occasions we had the worst of arguments.

As many readers may have predicted, after less than a week, we got back together on the agreement I'd move into my own place on my return to Australia where we could continue as a couple in separate homes. We then managed to enjoy the rest of our sunny holiday, trekking through rainforests, frolicking on beaches and dining on the ubiquitous seafood. Costa Rican vegetation has many versions of deep-green accentuated by the colours of sunsets, exotic plants and ocean views. Our photos feature wildlife: monkeys, tapirs, racoons, hummingbirds, giant turtles and those glorious slow-moving sloths (in Spanish *perezosos,* or lazy ones).

Luke and I have different travelling styles. He's highly organised and likes every detail planned in advance after a thorough risk analysis. I'm happy to travel like this in high season, but in low season, when crowds aren't a problem, I'd rather be spontaneous and leave things to chance. I can't say my heart was heavy when we parted ways after three weeks. Now I was free to make things up as I went along and follow my whims. My first impulse was to settle for a week and attend a Spanish language school.

When I turned up for my first day at school, in the tiny, Afro-Caribbean beach town of Puerto Viejo, I learned that I'd be the only person in my class. In fact, I'd be the only person in the whole school, which turned out to be fully outdoor: an overgrown field with a sheltered kitchen, hammock and a couple of tables. To convince me it was a school, there was a small whiteboard on a stand.

I met my teacher, a father of three who kept applying lavender oil to his wrists to sniff. This was to self-soothe: his dog had died the previous night and he felt stressed about breaking the news to his three little daughters later that day. I'd been surprised that the Costa Ricans I'd met, predominantly men, had anglicised names like Dennis, Henry and Walter. My Spanish teacher's name was Elmer. I wondered if I'd meet more Costa Rican women before my trip ended and whether their names might be more Spanish.

To my surprise, Elmer was writing a book that touched on plant medicines, although his was a biography of an aging American surfer known as Captain Zero, who'd settled in Puerto Viejo after he'd served time in gaol in the US for decades of marijuana trafficking. He in turn was surprised to learn that I was also writing a book, on psychedelics. Elmer and I would have plenty to talk about, albeit in Spanish, which was hard work at my low level. Elmer had taken magic mushrooms when he was 25, which led him to quit smoking. He'd been a heavy smoker since the age of seventeen with no intention of quitting but after taking the mushrooms he lost all desire to smoke.

Staying at the youth hostel across the road from the school (I was more than double everyone else's age but I had to cut costs), I met a young Dutch woman whose brother had taken ayahuasca. She told me he'd described his experience as 'having sex with the earth'.

Meeting the group

In the weeks leading up to the retreat, I'd developed a vision of my fellow retreatants: three earnest surfers from the United States, a couple of Europeans with rich backgrounds in psychedelics, a woman my age who might become a lifelong friend, and some form of an Australian, given Australians turn up everywhere. As with my past two retreats, we'd all bond beautifully over our shared interest in plant medicine, travel and learning. On the bus to the airport, where we were all to meet for the drive to the retreat centre, I could barely contain my excitement. I was about to meet some kindred spirits.

As it turned out, there would be only two other retreatants, a man and a woman from different parts of the state of Florida in the US. Our attempts to use WhatsApp to meet up at the airport proved stressful. In the interests of confidentiality, I'll spare the details, but suffice it to say that tempers frayed, things were said that could not be unsaid, and before we knew it our group was in a state of bitter conflict. We eventually piled into our car, over an hour late, for a tense drive to the healing centre. I felt like a character in a sitcom about incompatible people forced to spend time together.

On arrival, the hosts Carlos and Fanny greeted us warmly and showed us to our cabins separately. This gave each of us an opportunity to vent to them about our *compañeros*. Carlos spent almost an hour talking to each person separately to understand what they brought to this retreat, after which he worked his magic to reconcile us and set us up for the retreat:

> While our retreat groups are usually six-to-nine people, this group, by sheer chance, was going to be four but someone got COVID, so now you are three. You have to realise that it's not a coincidence that you three have been thrown together. We attract people into our lives that rub us the wrong way so that we can learn. I want you to see each other as teachers. What can each person show me about myself? You'll learn from each other's experiences as well—all the learning can be shared in a collective consciousness. When I heal, you heal, and vice versa.

At least, with only three of us, we'd all get a room to ourselves.

Carlos

Carlos had left Costa Rica for a career in New York where he worked for five years as an electrical engineer before returning to Costa Rica to start his own engineering business. He worked too hard, drank regularly with his basketball and business buddies, ate badly, became overweight and has a photo to prove it.

Over a period of nine years, his sister struggled with cancer and at the age of 31 passed away, leaving deep scars on Carlos. Around this time, he started to see that his goal in life was to be better than others, to be the best in every endeavour, but also that none of this was making him the slightest bit happy. Even worse, he felt like he was living other people's lives rather than his own: conforming to others' expectations of him. He knew he needed to forge his own path and discover what he was supposed to do with his life.

One day, a childhood friend reappeared in his life, after an absence, and told Carlos: 'I've taken ayahuasca and I received a message: Carlos needs to take this medicine.'

On Carlos's first ayahuasca trip his deceased sister appeared to him and told him, 'I died for you, Carlos. Make sure you go and give love to people.' She shared her knowledge with him and taught him about 'energy' and 'vibration' and helped him to see what he needed to do with his life.

Carlos continued to take ayahuasca with a shaman and was constantly amazed at how much it taught him. Sometimes a trip would leave him feeling that now he knew everything, but his next trip would only teach him how little he knew. In the earlier days of taking ayahuasca, he was still trapped in an unhealthy lifestyle of eating and drinking carelessly and of being the person others demanded him to be, but cracks were not only appearing, they were blasting open. His business fell over, leaving him with over $300,000 of debt. A business partner betrayed him. His marriage ended. Then he had an ayahuasca trip that would wake him, once and for all, from the slumber.

Carlos died.

He'd taken some ayahuasca and it felt like every organ in his body shut down. His heartbeat galloped and he felt as sick as a body can feel. He rang the shaman who'd provided the medicine and told him, 'I've had a heart attack, help me', but the shaman replied, 'If this is your time to go then there's nothing anyone can do for you'. Carlos found himself in a place of blackness, where nothing existed, he stayed there for what felt like eternity—although it was probably a couple of hours in earth time.

A feminine divinity finally appeared and took Carlos in her arms. Cradling him like a baby she whispered in his ear, 'Don't waste your life again'.

Now Carlos had the impetus to commit to making dramatic changes to his lifestyle and taking his first steps on the path of sharing ayahuasca with others. This was the work he believed he was supposed to do, and he started running retreats.

Carlos had been running retreats for about five years when he joined up with Fanny and they found their current retreat site, which was available for rent. It was completely dilapidated but had a stupendous view. Carlos saw the potential but he needed to rebuild the main house and build an accommodation block for retreatants. He didn't have the money but fate would provide. He'd lent money to a woman in need and eventually she rang him and said she was able to pay him back. As he drove to her house, the GPS took him the wrong way and as he reversed back along a narrow road, part of the road was unstable and his car tumbled over a cliff. It somersaulted down into a river where it began to fill with water. Someone must have seen it happen as the ambulance and fire brigade arrived soon to rescue him. Carlos was extracted from his written-off car completely unharmed. His rescuers advised him to go straight to hospital, but he knew there was no need. A few weeks later, he received an insurance payout that would finance the renovation of the new retreat centre. On his road to establishing his retreats, Carlos found that bizarre coincidences like this kept occurring.

Fanny

Fanny started her career as an interpreter and translator of English. Overly dedicated, she became a workaholic who failed to look after herself physically, but her biggest problem was that she lived in chronic pain. She went from doctor to doctor but her tests always came back suggesting no problems. One doctor even scolded her for wasting his time.

She started studying holistic medicine and learned how to detoxify her body by nourishing it with healthy food. She went from seeing a doctor three times a week to not needing to see a doctor for the last fifteen years.

Her studies of holistic medicine led her to open her own clinic and also lead retreats for cancer patients, teaching them how to nourish and heal themselves. So many who attended had been told they only had a few months or years left to live. Fanny was stunned by how many of them, after attending her retreats, lived far longer than predicted or were even healed altogether.

Fanny had been part of a group that pooled their funds to pay for a shaman to come from South America every year to run an ayahuasca ceremony, and for a few years she benefitted from an annual ceremony. Motivated by a sense that something was missing in her life, she eventually learned that what she was looking for had been inside her all along.

One day Fanny gave a talk at a conference about healing from cancer and Carlos was in the audience. They struck up a friendship based on common interests, especially their shared interest in healing. Carlos was still married at that time so there had been nothing romantic in their relationship. Before long, Carlos said to Fanny, 'When I eventually have a large retreat centre, I'd love to offer you a job.'

'Why wait until you have a large retreat centre?' Fanny asked. 'I've got experience starting new ventures.'

So they started working together, holding ceremonies and running their healing centre. Through their work over the years, they gradually grew closer and became a couple.

As the retreats became more established, attracting people from all over the world, Carlos was approached by someone with money who suggested they join forces and run bigger retreats. He turned it down. By that stage both Fanny and Carlos loved running small retreats where they could connect deeply with each participant.

13

First ayahuasca ceremony

FANNY GAVE US A tour of the property, which was perched on a mountaintop. A two-storey house opened onto a giant patio where a built-in pool had been filled with concrete, creating space for a fire cauldron for retreatants to sit around. A row of banana chairs looked out on the rolling mountain view. As we walked down the steep hill from the house, we saw the two teepees where I assumed our trips would take place. I took many photos of the trees on the property as I'd never seen bark that looked like impressionist paintings with dabs of pink, spearmint green, white and burnt orange. Sprawling tree roots created foot-traps for the unwary.

Fanny's introductory talk to the three of us came to me as a series of shocks. I knew that the three ayahuasca ceremonies would be at night but I'd assumed they would start in the evening.

'Just go to bed in the evening when you're tired and we'll wake you up late at night and take you to the teepee for the ceremony.'

Only a fellow insomniac could understand the alarm this triggered in me. On this seven-night retreat, I could count on at least three sleepless nights. On the positive side, sleep deprivation brings out the worst in me and this could be useful. What better way to bring out your shadow side so that Mama Ayahuasca could work on it?

'Do ayahuasca ceremonies always have to be at night?' I queried.

'You need complete darkness to get the full effect of the visuals,' replied Fanny.

'Of course,' I nodded.

Just when I thought things couldn't become any more difficult, Fanny added another detail.

'You'll eat breakfast on the day of the ceremony but after that you'll need to fast for the rest of the day. This helps you vomit less.'

I've never been into fasting even though some people swear by it as a means for spiritual openings. I eat more than a lot of men I know. Usually I cope with sleep-deprivation by eating, which boosts my mood and energy levels. This week, I would not only be sleep-deprived, but also hungry. This retreat was not going to be a picnic. I made a mental note to be grateful for the climate: after the heat and humidity of the coast, the cool mountain air and constant sunshine provided some comfort.

Finally, I knew we would need to surrender our phones and laptops and I'd been looking forward to switching off from the outside world, but we'd also need to surrender our watches. I'm so addicted to checking the time every few minutes I knew I'd feel completely unmoored.

A characteristic this retreat would share with the Buddhist retreats I'd attended was the opportunity to spend many hours alone with the mind. Unlike Natasja's retreats, there was a minimal program of activities. Fanny told me that they often veto applicants aged in their twenties for fear that many of them aren't mature enough to cope without a schedule.

'Keep in mind,' Fanny continued, 'that all three ceremonies are likely to be completely different for you. You'll also have different experiences to each other and it's best to avoid comparing experiences, which is never helpful.'

'I've never taken any illegal drugs in my life,' said one of the Floridians. 'So I have to admit, I'm a bit nervous.'

'You can trust,' replied Fanny, 'that ayahuasca won't give you anything you can't handle. Some people describe ayahuasca as an *abuela*—the grandmother who takes the child by the hand and shows her scenes from her life that she can learn from.'

'Remember too,' Fanny added, 'that the medicine itself is not what changes you. Integration afterwards can be more important than the medicine itself, so put your focus on integration—talk to us after your ceremony. Be in touch with your feelings and your body sensations. Rest. Of course, the best thing for integration is sleep.'

Great.

Excursion to the conservation forest and rapeh

The five of us piled into a car and took a scenic drive through the greenest of mountains. I got into journalist mode and picked Fanny's brain.

'What have you found is the most common reason that people come on your retreats?' I asked.

'There are two main reasons. People either want to address trauma from their childhood, or they want to deepen their spiritual practice.'

'Do your retreats attract more men or women?'

'For the first few years they seemed to attract more women but since COVID we've seen more men coming through. The trend reversed.'

'Is there anything in particular you've found surprising over the years?'

'I've witnessed with men,' Carlos answered, 'that the tougher they present, the more likely they are to be crying on the floor like a baby during the ceremony. We had a retreatant once from the mafia. We didn't realise he was from the mafia and he'd actually stopped his mafia involvement shortly before the retreat. He cried a lot. And then we had a professional fighter who also cried a lot. He had a flashback doing ayahuasca where he saw himself as a three-year-old boy watching his mother being beaten up. He'd felt helpless and realised that addressing that feeling was the reason he'd been a fighter all his life.'

After about half an hour's drive, we arrived at their private forest. Carlos told us they'd only just bought it using the proceeds from the retreats. 'The money you paid for this retreat is helping to support this beautiful forest,' he told us. It was also the place they were planning to move their retreats in two years when their lease ran out on the current centre.

Carlos told us to wander slowly along the trail, a few metres between each other, while he and Fanny would drive to the other end to meet us. For half an hour we strolled through, taking it all in. How pleasant it was to have permission to move slowly. I'd been travelling for weeks in Costa Rica, visiting many forests and jungles, but this one was the most beautiful, probably because of the moss growing here, which made the trees look dressed up in fluffy clothes. It was primary forest, dense, diverse, with a mysterious magical quality. I was mindful of plant intelligence, so often raised in the psychedelic literature, and felt the trees communing with me, a feeling I'd had around trees for some months now.

When we arrived at the clearing, Carlos announced a rapeh ceremony. I remembered taking rapeh at the Bufo retreat where it had made me feel still and present. First, we'd each be shamanically 'cleaned' as Fanny took a smoking pot of burning sage round the perimeter of our bodies. Carlos blew some rapeh powder up our noses, both nostrils, in order that we ingest it properly. Like having half a jar of paprika whooshed up your nose, it wasn't pleasant. My eyes watered and my sinuses stung as I coughed and wiped tears from my face.

Once the unpleasantness passed, I looked up at a small tree in front of me and felt it love me. I placed my hand lovingly on my cheek and repeated, '*mi cariño*', Spanish for 'my dear'. From that point, I felt effortlessly mindful of my body and its every sensation.

Rapeh sessions are over quickly and a few minutes later we headed back to the retreat centre. The rapeh had made me feel lethargic as though I'd had too much to drink. I thought to myself, *Well the trippy part was nice but not quite worth the initial discomfort and this lethargy. I don't think I'll do it again.*

Alas, I would.

Preparation talk before the first ceremony

It would be a lie to say this is the preparation talk Carlos gave before the first ceremony. He gave this talk as preparation before *every* ceremony, as integration *after* every ceremony, and in most of his one-to-one chats with me. Of course, he'd provide different examples to demonstrate his point, but he was always on message. I'd catch myself thinking, 'He's a qualified engineer with a brilliant mind, fascinated by science and so many different topics, yet this is what he talks about, two retreats a month, so many times on every retreat. Doesn't he get bored by the repetition? Doesn't he want to explore other topics?' Yet every time Carlos gave his talk it seemed he couldn't be happier, as though he was saying it for the first time in his life.

This was the talk:

> Keep asking yourself, during the ceremony, during your day, whatever you're doing: Who is experiencing this?
>
> Who is eating this sandwich? Who is thinking this thought? Who is feeling this emotion?

> We're all on a journey to discover our true selves. None of us are who we think we are. So find out who you are. One way is to determine who you're not. With investigation you'll discover you're not your job—you might lose your job, but you will still be you. You're not your roles—roles can change over our lifetime, one day I'm a son, then I'm a father and then a grandfather. You're not your body—even if you became a quadriplegic, you'd still be you. You are not your thoughts—thoughts just vanish after you think them.
>
> So what's left? Consciousness.
>
> The small mind will constantly try to tell you who you are but the mind is wrong. The mind is a beautiful and helpful instrument, but it can't tell you who you are. Of course, you'll never be able to stop the mind and its chattering, but don't let it fool you. Learn to observe it and not believe it.

When we'd share our hang-ups and difficulties, no matter what they were, Carlos would not become entangled in details but, rather, would say, 'Ask yourself, who's telling you that? It's just the mind, it's not the real you.' Sometimes he'd say, 'That's coming from the *little* you.'

So the answer to 'Who's experiencing this?' in any given moment, is either going to be 'the mind', the little me, or consciousness. In Buddhism, they refer to consciousness as 'pure awareness' or 'the unconditioned', but Carlos will tell you that every spiritual tradition has its equivalent. Christianity has the Holy Spirit or the Soul. Some call it the Beloved, the Divine or God.

Carlos's talk usually finished with the words:

> Once we realise, on the deepest level, that we are not our mind, that we are more than our thoughts, our roles, our body or our possessions, it brings everything in our lives into question. We find that we need to start all over again.

I was surprised when Carlos told me he'd never read a Buddhist book in his life. A past retreatant had given him one as a gift but he'd only dipped into it, now and then, and had never read it from cover to cover.

'But everything you teach comes straight from Buddhism,' I blurted. 'Observe your thoughts. Don't identify with them. Question the illusion of having a self. It's all Buddhism!'

'All the major religions of the world,' Carlos said, 'are just the finger pointing at the moon, not the moon itself. In the same way, none of the religions are the truth itself but a way to reach the truth. They all lead to the same place.'

Carlos took from all spiritual traditions, not attaching to any particular one. The retreat centre is decorated with iconography from all the main traditions, with most of the décor—the books, ornaments and wall-hangings—gifts from past retreatants.

Carlos's approach chimes with that of Stanislav Grof's, the 'Godfather of LSD' and inventor of Holotropic Breathwork who wrote:

> A deep mystical experience tends to dissolve the boundaries between religions and reveals deep connections between them, while dogmatism of organised religions tends to emphasize differences between various creeds and engender antagonism and hostility.[1]

Grof also speaks of how psychedelics help us develop:

> '. . . a spirituality of universal and mystical nature that—unlike faith in the dogmas of mainstream religions—is authentic and convincing, since it is based on deep personal experience.'

I can't help thinking that such an approach might contribute to more world peace.

Trip one

I assumed the three ceremonies would take place in a teepee but there was yet another larger rectangular tent hidden at the bottom of the sloping property and this one had enough space to hold a party for fifty. The candlelit room was a sight to behold, its walls decorated with spiritual symbolism from all the main traditions. At the entryway Fanny 'cleansed' us, one by one, taking the pot of smoking sage round our bodies. We each had a mattress to lie on, with a pillow and two blankets.

Fanny and Carlos sat cross-legged at the front and the three of us left our mattresses to gather close to them in a small circle. Carlos explained to us:

> Ayahuasca works through symbols so don't bother trying to make sense of them during the trip. Their meaning may become clear at some point in the future, maybe the next day, maybe years later. There's nothing you have to do: just lie there and surrender to it. If the thinking mind tries to get involved,

just observe it, don't let it take over. Your mind will keep doing its thing in the background, trying to interpret and make sense of the experience, but you'll notice that when the mind interferes, the experience often disappears altogether.

It may help to focus on the music, which can anchor you in the experience.

Drink the medicine fast. It's not pleasant but you can take some ginger and honey straight afterwards.

He performed shamanic rituals with smoke and glowing sticks that looked like cigars. He made patterns in the air with the glowing stick and blew smoke on each of us.

One by one, we sat in front of Carlos to receive the medicine in a sacred moment: he prayed over the cup before placing it in my hands, then covering my hands with his, we sat silently for a few seconds in stillness. Not only did the medicine taste vile but it felt like trying to swallow a heavily powdered liquid. It was hard not to gag.

The three of us went to lie on our mattresses and donned our eye masks. After what felt like twenty minutes the show began.

I see the word 'gentleness' up in lights and images appear, one after the next, all profoundly beautiful. These are the most enchanting images I've ever seen, even better than the psilocybin visuals. They take me by surprise with their complexity and brilliance and I'm in awe as my body dissolves to merge with each scene. Why do people go travelling the world when you can see all this lying in one place? Marek has to do this. Luke has to do this—he wouldn't believe it.

I feel welcomed by Mama Ayahuasca—I feel her deep love and care for me and how she wants to make me welcome with all this gentleness. The music from the playlist fuels my euphoria and my body resumes all the usual shuddering, shaking, yawns, quiet moans, stomach clenching and sudden sit-ups.

Now I'm in a theme park, with a pastel colour theme, full of merry-go-rounds and choo-choo trains, all the rides move exceptionally slowly—is this a message that I need more slow time in my life? I try to talk to the cartoonish humans, all plump and cheerful, but I struggle to produce language. They don't understand me anyway. I start a sentence several times but can't get any words out. I approach a sweet cartoon lady on a choo-choo train and try to speak. Smiling and shaking her head, she waves a hand as if to say, 'I don't speak English' but what she means is, 'We don't need language here, don't bother trying'.

I feel deeply happy at this theme park, an unconditional happiness, not based on anything in particular happening. I'm happy because, in some way, I'm home.

All at once, I'm not at the theme park anymore but in a series of jewel-studded environments beyond all description. The mind repeatedly asks, How could I ever convey any of this in writing? So many sights I've never seen before. Out of nowhere, I hear words from a man with an Australian accent: 'You can hang around and enjoy this place for ages, but you can't take anything with you.' I know he's right and that I'll only vaguely remember a couple of images.

I feel an intermittent nausea and would welcome a vomit to relieve it but can't seem to bring anything up.

A female presence appears, she's two-dimensional, composed of a few geometric shapes. She hovers above me, looking down and I feel her loving presence strongly: I commune with her, marvel at her realness and how close she feels to me. Sometimes she has some helpers who understand that my body feels cold: they cover me with blankets and stroke and soothe me. The Divine Feminine comes closer and I feel her pressing two fingers down on either side of my hips. I wonder if she's healing them of their arthritic tendencies.

I travel again to a new realm, beyond my ability to describe, where I notice that all the parts of my body are separated, existing in several different locations. I ask: Who is experiencing this? Who am I now? I am a disembodied head. That is who is experiencing this: my severed head. I am, therefore, not my body. And without my body parts, what's left? Only consciousness of my present moment. That's who I am.

Integration with Carlos

I must've fallen asleep at the end of the trip, for when I woke up, the others had all left the room. Only Carlos remained and he sat next to me and asked how I was feeling.

'Great. Wow. Even now, though, straight after the trip, I can't remember the details of most of the beautiful views I saw,' I lamented.

'There's a part of you that does remember, your soul. You'll always have them,' Carlos replied.

I tell Carlos about the God-like woman I met.

'Even though I had an encounter with the Divine Feminine, I feel like there should be more of a sense of "wow" but I feel underwhelmed for some reason.'

'Who is saying there should be a feeling of "wow"? That's the little you, the mind.'

'I guess it shows the mind can't always be trusted: I meet God, or God-*ess*, but my mind fails to react appropriately. I noticed that thoughts, or inner chatter, still came up throughout the trip—like the mind just won't stop no matter what's going on.'

'It happens during trips as it happens in life. The mind will never stop producing its endless thoughts and judgements. Just observe it and remember that it's not necessarily right and it's not who you are.'

Since I had Carlos to myself, I took the opportunity to raise another topic even though it didn't arise in my trip.

'How have you coped with the issue of losing friends throughout your life?' I spring on him.

Carlos took a moment to collect his thoughts.

'I realised that the friends I had in my life before ayahuasca all wanted something from me, and that's not true friendship. When I gave up going to bars to drink with friends, I lost all my drinking friends. When I closed down my business, I lost all my business friends.'

'So how did that make you feel to lose all those friends?' I asked.

'Beautiful,' he replied. I flinched at the unexpected answer.

'Didn't you feel sad, and alone, to lose all your friends? And it happened to you twice! Doesn't that leave a huge gap in your life that's just . . . not filled?'

'I'd moved to a new vibrational frequency where I could be there to love myself. Losing friends is part of life's journey. You start on a new path. You make new friends.'

I quibbled with him for a while but ultimately admired his resilience and flexible perspective.

Sitting in the banana chairs overlooking the rolling mountain view, the two Floridians and I shared details of our trips and marvelled at how different they all were.

Carlos was right: these two were great teachers. They didn't turn out to be the people I expected them to be when I first met them. They both continued to surprise me and make me question first impressions. When you get to know people who seem completely different to yourself and hear their backstories, compassion is the only response. Within a couple of days, the three of us were fond of each other. Whether we sat around a fire, admired a sunset, or sat in silence together, we began to feel like a close-knit family. We'd even stay in touch long after the retreat ended.

14

Second ayahuasca ceremony

As THE DAYS PASSED, I took long walks up and down the mountain, or found lookouts from which to gaze for hours at the stunning mountain ranges. It helped that the weather was perfect every day: sunny and mild. It was the rainy season but the rain only lasted an hour, at the most. I meditated, journalled and chatted, occasionally, with the Floridians. I also needed to spend whole days in bed as my body recovered from the trials of fasting, sleep deprivation and the ayahuasca ceremonies, which made me feel as heavy as concrete and utterly unable to be upright.

Carlos and Fanny were always around and you could have a chat to them whenever you felt like it. They had no need for personal boundaries and seemed to thoroughly enjoy their chats with us, even seek them out. I'm experienced with retreats, Buddhist and now plant medicine retreats, and knew that retreatants always made an appointment with the teachers, usually for a fifteen-minute chat. I would soon have a chat with Fanny that went for two hours.

I asked Carlos if their high availability was because there were only three of us.

'No,' he replied, 'we don't use a schedule for integration even when there's eight or nine.'

Carlos agreed when I suggested this was another reason they wanted to keep retreat numbers low.

The second rapeh ceremony

The night after the first ayahuasca ceremony I obviously needed a good night's sleep, but I woke to the noise of a distant dog barking. On and on. Without a watch I had no idea what time it was but I tossed and turned for hours. I was so disappointed by my burgeoning sleep deficit. When it goes too far, my mood can plummet, and there would be evidence of this the next day.

We assembled in the trip-tent, in the afternoon, unsure why, but it turned out to be for another rapeh ceremony.

Shit.

I didn't feel like it but couldn't quite bring myself to say so. Why was I such a pleaser? Why couldn't I find my voice? I knew they wouldn't force me if I spoke up but I couldn't find my voice. I filled with dread. I'm so weak at tolerating physical discomfort. I just want to feel nice and comfortable all the time. That's the kind of person I am. But it was my turn and Carlos blew the powdery substance up my nose.

Pwof!

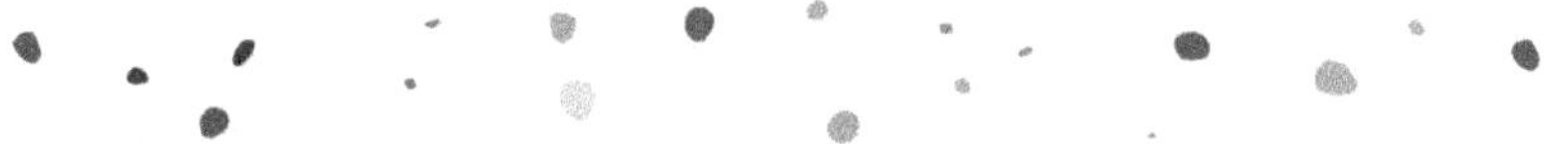

Pain is my teacher. Pain is my teacher. Pain is my teacher. I hate, hate, hate this.

I weep, defeated. But resistance is futile. Slowly the discomfort fades and I hear the line from the hymn:

BE STILL AND KNOW THAT I AM GOD.

Hmm, what's that all about?

Next a string of random memories from the past assails me: Alex latching on to my breast after being born; the worst thing my husband ever said to me; lying in bed with a long-running illness; letting down my oldest friend. And then I think: am I going to fail this retreat and not learn who I truly am? How many years practising Buddhism did I fail to realise who I am, without my ego?

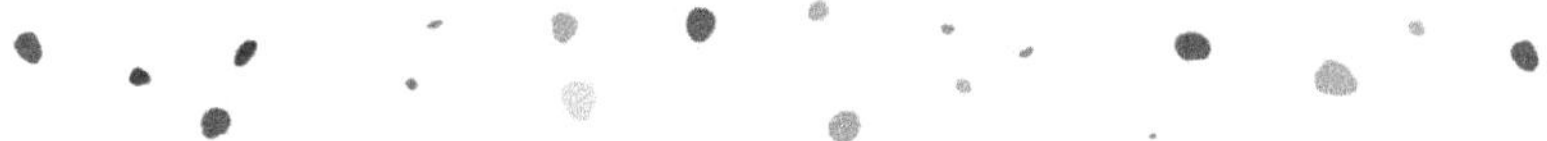

We go around the group to share what just happened for us but I'm not in the mood and I feel upset. I start ugly crying in front of the group as I blather: 'I just don't know if I'm going to have the breakthrough and realise, deeply, who is experiencing this, who I am. I've grappled with this teaching for decades. I've read the books. I've even written a few about it but I feel like I only really understand it at the conceptual level and not on a deeper level. Not in my heart. I'm hearing at this retreat—and I received a strong message from my trip—to leave language behind, that this is a word-free zone. But language is my medium, it's how I operate.'

'You just need to connect the conceptual understanding with your heart,' replied Carlos.

'But I don't want to waste more time chasing ego death. I don't want to feel like I've failed the retreat when I don't get it,' I sobbed and sniffled.

'But you've already got it. It's already there.'

'You speak in riddles,' I said, almost aggressively.

'For me,' Carlos shared, 'my ego dissolved one day when I was staring into the eyes of my dog.'

This might sound a little dubious, but believe me, Carlos's German shepherd, Roff, is some kind of spiritual being. Staring into Roff's eyes is quite an experience. He does receive regular acupuncture for arthritis, which might give him a spiritual edge.

The other two retreatants shared their experiences and when everyone filed out Fanny stayed behind with me for a chat.

She looked me in the eye with her warm smile and shook her head: 'I understand you so deeply, Sarah.'

I don't think anyone's ever said that to me before.

'When it comes to books and learning and collecting knowledge,' she explained 'I've been on the same journey as you. I had four qualifications and I loved studying and book-learning. I knew, though, that to do the work I do now, working with people on retreats, I needed to learn to engage with people from a deeper part of myself. I was so used to helping people using my book knowledge—that was how I connected, how I related to my patients and all the people I met. But I needed to learn to connect with people from my heart, to speak to them from that place, from my true nature and it was a really hard lesson for me. In my clinic I had all my qualifications and certificates framed on the wall and I felt so proud of them. They were who I was! It was a painful transition to detach from all that and engage with people from a deeper place inside myself. I knew there needed to be a marriage of the mind and the heart where the mind always bowed to the heart.

'I had an ayahuasca trip,' Fanny continued, 'where I threw all my certificates, for all my qualifications, on a fire. It was painful to do but I knew it was necessary. I told Carlos about the trip and that I wanted to throw my real certificates on a fire as well but Carlos suggested I wait: "You've done it on an energetic level and that's more important than the physical level". So I collected them all into a box and moved them into storage at my mother's place and forgot about them. Years later, I was rummaging through some boxes and found the one with my qualifications. When I found that box, I was amazed to observe that I felt nothing. There was a time when looking at those certificates was such an emotional experience of pride and satisfaction but now, nothing—and that felt good. I said to my nephew who was with me at the time that I was probably going to throw them out and he raised his eyebrows and said, "What if you need it for a future job?" I just laughed. I was running ayahuasca retreats by then and said, "I'll never want another job".'

I return to my room and suddenly feel embarrassed. I'd cried—blathered—in front of a group. *You've just behaved like a fucking idiot*, I say to myself. Who cries about failing to achieve ego dissolution? I could barely recognise myself. It's not as though it's something I worry about in my daily life.

It so happened, though, that the rapeh experience set me up for the next ayahuasca trip.

Trip two

For my second trip, two nights later, I felt like I drank double what I drank the previous ceremony and I could not finish drinking the foul liquid without gagging. I needed to pause and recover before I could finish the dose. In this trip I would experience Mama Ayahuasca as the *abuela*, the grandmother holding my hand, guiding me through some spiritual truths. Eight scenes from among scores of images were available to my memory when it was over.

Again, the exquisite images. They seem so familiar while I'm in the trip, yet I know I won't remember them. Except one: I look out over a vast valley of pure whiteness, filled with bejewelled palaces and objects of extreme beauty. I perceive a message: All this comes from inside you, it's all within you, you have everything you need, honour the Divine in yourself.

•

Through some strange symbols and images, I perceive a new sense of who I am: a me without my baggage, a me who has let go of her history—all the past rejections, any feelings of not belonging, or not feeling cared for. It's all gone and the new me feels light and free.

Suddenly, I vomit. It's like a tennis ball of black tar and sludge. Released. It was my ego. Gone, for good.

Now I'm a hybrid octopus-alien, made out of seaweed, talking to another similar creature. We hang from wires that are part of a network of chairlifts over a huge valley. The other alien yells:

'SARAH IS GONE.'

'What a relief,' alien-me replies, laughing, 'I was tired of looking after her.'

The other alien repeats it a few times with jubilation as though some dreadful dictator's reign has finally ended:

'SARAH IS GONE.'

I'm excited and ready to live life without all the stories I cling to about who I am. No more living in reaction to the past.

●

'Me' has transformed into another creature who shudders violently as life energy pours into me, and onto its next destination: I'm an essential part of a complex network of energy flow.

I now understand that my ongoing shuddering in daily life is spiritual and binds me to the energy flow of the spirit world.

●

Now I see many images of my son Alex. My love for him is so strong that I'm sobbing with the force of it. Sobbing from love, though, soon turns to sobbing with grief, the tears of a mother who has watched her son suffer for several years. I cry hard and it feels good to release the tears. I hold him tight. I love him so much. It's a beautiful feeling, but also painful.

As I promised Alex before I left home, I interrogate the medicine, 'Is there a message for Alex?' The answer comes immediately: 'He carries not only his own pain but also intergenerational trauma.' I see an image of Alex lying in a narrow stream, through which the energy of suffering flows, the suffering of all the people who share similar trials in life to him, but also the suffering that comes from unresolved family traumas through the generations, especially those from the war-ravaged land of Poland. He was born into this energy stream.

●

As happened on my Bufo trip, I revisit my old bedroom again, where I lie depressed, mentally inflicting physical harm on myself. A hybrid insect-bird lands next to my ear and says, 'Why couldn't you be there for yourself? Why would you willingly add to your pain by being cruel to yourself? You have to BE THERE FOR YOU when you're hurting.'

●

I see Luke lying in his bed alone, without me. Is he lonely? My heart opens. He is no longer merely a problem to solve but a precious human being. I snuggle up to him and send him lovingkindness.

●

I revisit a childhood memory. I was in first grade, at school, and left the classroom to retrieve something from my 'tote-tray' in the next room. The simple action of pulling my tray out somehow triggered a heavy box to fall from above me and it crashed to the floor creating an almighty mess. The noise was loud and gave me a tremendous fright.

The teacher, Miss Black, ran into the room to see what the commotion was. Seeing the mess on the floor, she looked into my eyes with a face full of contempt and said, 'You're a very naughty girl.' I was a first grader. I wanted to be a good girl, not a naughty girl. I re-experience the shame and now see what is triggered in my daily life when I feel someone might be even the slightest bit angry with me.

A disembodied head appears. It looks like a man in his early sixties but I understand it to be the Holy Spirit for it says, 'Who do you think has been here all along with you? I knew about the crying Baby Sarah who you met doing MDMA. Who else could know about this?'

Excellent point. It hits me: there must be something other than my mind that could access that lost memory from my infancy that plagued my psilocybin trip and became clarified in my MDMA trip.

'Shouldn't you be female?' I ask, but he whooshes away, out of sight.

All the same, now I feel the 'wow'. Strong evidence for the Divine within.

Integration with Fanny

Again, I must've fallen asleep towards the end of my experience and when I awoke the other retreatants had left. Fanny lay on a mattress across the tent with her eyes open. She must've been waiting for hours for me to wake up. Carlos and Fanny would never leave a retreatant alone to stumble back up the hill on their own. Fanny then spent almost two hours with me discussing the trip and other life matters.

'How are you feeling?' Fanny asked.

'Extremely exhausted like I've been hit by a bus, but it was a really amazing trip,' I replied.

I shared with Fanny the scene where the seaweed octopus-alien announces, 'Sarah Is Gone'. In those early moments after the trip, I did believe that my ego had been defeated once and for all.

'How does that feel for you right now?' Fanny asked.

'I feel really free and light and spacious and optimistic about the future,' I declared, believing that this was the new me.

'Just remember, that whatever happens, there will always be a pattern of Expansion-Contraction-Expansion-Contraction. That's just life.'

It would only take a few more hours to realise that my ego, my sense of a 'self' and its baggage to lug around, was still in place. Still, I'd probably released some of it, just not all of it. Like the Buddhist teacher Jack Kornfield wrote in *After the Ecstasy, the Laundry*: 'There's no enlightened retirement.'[1]

'When I vomited,' I told Fanny, 'I felt like I'd vomited my ego out. I never imagined vomiting could be a symbol.'

'That makes sense to me,' replied Fanny. 'Once I'd taken mescaline, which led to a full night of vomiting—and I mean hours and hours of it. It's an unusual reaction to mescaline but it can happen. It forms a jelly in your gut, which is really difficult to purge, so the vomiting is really hard work and I spent that night hugging the toilet, in extreme discomfort. And yet, Sarah, I felt grateful through the whole experience. Gratitude doesn't only have to be for the pleasant, joyful moments in life. Even the bad moments are teaching us things we need to learn and for that we can feel grateful and I'm telling you, I felt grateful that night with every fibre of my being. I even felt grateful for feeling grateful and I have felt grateful for everything, good and bad, ever since.'

I doubted I'd ever reach Fanny's level of spiritual development.

Predictably, I started talking to Fanny about my ailing relationship only to find she'd had a similar relationship in the past, for ten years, so understood my issues perfectly.

'I feel so unbearably guilty,' I began, 'when I disappoint others, when I can't be what they want me to be, when I cause them to suffer. I need out of the relationship, but I'm scared to pull the trigger. I want to relieve suffering in the world, but all I seem to do is create more.'

'Sarah, you may cause a time of difficulty for a partner if you break up with them but that might be exactly what a partner needs in order to grow and learn the lessons they are supposed to learn in this lifetime. Sometimes you have to focus on what you need yourself to ensure that you are on the right path for you. If a relationship is not working for you, then you have to do the right thing for yourself. Besides, you can't predict what will happen for your partner—there are hundreds of possibilities, including finding a situation that makes him happier and including getting back together after you've both done some work on yourselves.

'Partners are mirrors,' she continued. 'Just as we need a physical mirror to check our hair and outfit, a partner provides the kind of mirror that enables you to see your flaws. Most people find it very difficult to accept their flaws so we project them onto the other person. Just as you would never use a comb on the mirror to fix your hair, nor can we fix ourselves by trying to change our partner.'

'So once your ten-year relationship finally ended, how did you cope with living on your own?' I asked.

'I love living on my own. It feels like a time for releasing attachments, to become more self-sufficient. I can be happy living alone, but also in a relationship, as I am now with Carlos. Either is fine for me. Living on my own I realised that if I ever shared my life again it would have to be with someone who is: a) conscious, and b) someone who would allow me the freedom to do the things I need to do.'

'I certainly enjoy *travelling* on my own. I'll try to remember the example set by you, and Carlos, when I return home to live on my own.'

'On another topic,' I continued, 'I feel like I'm learning a lot from the other two,' I said, referring to the Floridians, 'especially about how to feel love for people who are different from me. I think I have to admit that I've been a judgemental person from a young age. I've improved over time but I can be judgey during conversations with others always assessing the other person's conversational skills: do they "take turns" to speak, or do they talk *at* me? Do they listen? Do they take an interest in me or is it all about them? Are they long-winded and prone to waste my valuable time? Can they speak about anything other than their immediate world?'

Fanny nodded knowingly and said, 'Judgements always, always, always come from the small mind. When you notice that people aren't following your conversational rules you can remind yourself that we're all at a different point in our learning journey. You were once where they are. We're all operating at a different vibrational frequency.'

'But can't that be perceived as assuming I'm superior, to believe that people are at a lower vibrational frequency than me?'

'Not if you understand that they are you and you are them. Everybody is just a different part of yourself.'

I'd heard such a philosophy in Buddhism, but I felt on this retreat that it was becoming more than just a concept. I really did feel like the other two retreatants were me and I was them.

'I've also realised that I may be more advanced in some areas but not others,' I conceded. 'I've seen surprising kindness in one of them that I knew I would not have been capable of myself.'

I could think of many examples from my life of people who were poor in one area of psychological development but gifted in another. A Polish in-law came to mind. I used to resent her because she all but refused to speak to anyone on social occasions. It was as though she couldn't be bothered engaging. You'd ask her a question and she'd give you a one-word answer. Yet when the grandmother of the family got cancer and started to die, guess who was at her bedside all day, every day, tending to grandma's every need.

Temazcal in the sweat lodge

On one of my walks down the mountain outside the retreat centre, a car came to a stop beside me. I was relieved to see Fanny in her lemon-yellow mini.

'Jump in,' she said cheerfully.

'Oh,' I responded surprised. 'Was I supposed to be somewhere? What are we doing?'

'It's time for Temazcal in the sweat lodge,' Fanny replied.

'What's Temazcal? What's a sweat lodge?' I asked mildly flustered.

'You'll see,' Fanny replied with a grin.

Moments later, we arrived at the entry to a teepee and Fanny 'smudged' me, and the other retreatants, with the burning sage.

We all sat in the darkness of the teepee around a pile of rocks in the centre. Carlos told us the steps to this ceremony but my concentration was weak, due to my poor physical state. I felt overwhelmed, wishing I had the guts to ask him to repeat it all.

Next thing, Fanny asked me to open my mouth and emptied some powder into the side of my mouth, in front of my teeth, and told me to keep it there. 'Just swallow any liquid that is created,' she instructed. Then Carlos wiped something black and sticky on each of our hands—tobacco—and the instructions were to lick it from time to time. A worker came in and poured some liquid on the stones to make them heat up and before long we were sitting in a hot, steamy sauna in complete darkness.

'Think of anything you want to release into the heat,' instructed Carlos. 'Anything that's not serving you anymore.'

I thought about being a pleaser and my tendency to never rock the boat, to keep everyone happy no matter what the cost to myself. Especially in partner relationships. I'd try releasing some of that.

Soon enough, the steam made me feel heavy and exhausted. I could barely sit up, let alone keep my eyes open. In the darkness I could only just perceive someone place a maraca in one of my hands and a bongo drum in front of me and Carlos told us to make any noise we felt like. Before long, the small group was drumming a catchy rhythm, no doubt feeling connected, as though one. In the spirit of throwing away my pleaser tendencies, I messed up the group rhythm by drumming on the off beats, out of time and without any pattern. My contribution sounded awful, as though I was the black sheep in the group. I could imagine the others wondering, *What's* wrong *with her? Is she drunk or something?*, but I was grinning at my own mischief. It's fun to be a rebel sometimes, and next time I caught myself denying my needs in order to please others, I'd remember this scene.

15

Third ayahuasca ceremony

Given my exhaustion, I was in two minds about taking ayahuasca a third time. Carlos and Fanny had offered us the option of stopping after two ceremonies. While my body cried in desperation a big, fat 'no', I reasoned, 'Come on, you might never have the opportunity to take ayahuasca again. You've come all this way, made it this far. You don't want to spend the rest of your life wondering what a third trip would've revealed. Last night's trip was amazing. Do it!'

I remembered a different ayahuasca retreat I'd inquired about before settling on this one—I'd even done a Zoom interview with them, but that retreat was ten days and offered six ayahuasca ceremonies. I'd pulled out the moment before enrolling thinking six might be too many. I'd met psychonauts who spoke highly of such retreats but, personally, I lacked the stamina. I now thanked myself for making this decision as I struggled to commit to a third ceremony but, grudgingly, I would.

Lying in my bed for the hours before the ceremony started, hungry and sleep-deprived, my mood had turned toxic. I was full of dread for the nausea and possible vomiting ahead. When we finally took the steep track down to the tent, I couldn't have been grumpier. I lamented my mindset but hoped that, as with MDMA, it might not matter—but it would.

Once again, as I tried to drink the medicine I gagged before reaching the bottom of the cup. How I hated the ingestion. At least it only seemed to be a small dose tonight. I retired to my mattress to wait for the trip to start. I waited, however, for what seemed like a full hour, probably more. I knew I should've asked for a top-up of the medicine but I couldn't bring myself to drink any more of it.

Finally, some images begin to appear, but they are not the grand, magnificent visuals of my other trips. On the contrary, I seem to be in a community childcare centre in a poor neighbourhood. The colours seem faded, the images hazy, and I feel as though at a remove. Worse, although I have the image of the childcare centre in mind I don't feel as though I am anywhere other than lying on the mattress feeling just as cranky as I felt for the past few hours. Clearly, I haven't taken enough of the medicine to have a decent trip and yet I still have awful nausea leading to a particularly unpleasant vomit. Then a strong headache takes possession of me.

I lie there, critiquing the playlist and making a few attempts to get something started: 'I don't suppose I could talk to my late father?' I ask the medicine. No answer. 'Where's the Divine? Why can't something happen?' No answer.

At least I manage to escape the childcare centre for a new setting. I wander a grid of suburban streets but it all feels dreary. Huge primitive men roam the streets. For some reason, I know a lot of these men are paedophiles. I see a friend's husband grin at me and make the 'shh' sign in regard to an infidelity. I feel anxious in these streets for my sexual safety. As I move around town, sexualised images arise until I lose my patience. 'Not what I'm here for!' I murmur through gritted teeth.

Finally, the new day dawned but my crankiness had reached its peak. I sprang to my feet but felt so wobbly I knew I should not be up. I didn't care. I wanted to go to my proper bed. I faked sobriety and with Fanny's permission, wobbled back up the hill to return to my bed where I would spend the day nursing a strong headache, nausea and lethargy.

I wondered if I'd made the wrong decision to engage in the third ceremony. Or maybe my failure was being too lazy to ask for more medicine so that I could have a 'real trip'. Still, who knows? Sometimes, months or years later, a trip can make more sense, the meaning suddenly revealed. In this case though, I'd be surprised.

Group integration

One of the Floridians had experienced three trips resembling my third. Along with nausea and headaches she described her experiences: 'I'm not sure if I was even awake or the whole thing was a dream, but I only remember a couple of images and they don't make much sense—that's all I've got.' Yet the medicine must have done something for her if the 'before' and 'after' are anything to go by. When she first arrived, she was clearly weighed down by the troubles in her world—family conflicts, loneliness, health problems, a recent layoff from work. Yet the same woman, on leaving the retreat, couldn't have been more optimistic about the future. Her face looked different: there was a lightness and an openness to her expression. She smiled, and laughed, more easily. All her sentences started with, 'When I get home, I'm going to . . .' and then there'd be an inspiring resolution like, '. . . take up hiking' or, '. . . detoxify my body' or 'apply for that other job'.

The other Floridian was a man of few words but it was clear he was leaving way happier than the lost soul I'd met on the first day. Extremely fit and half my age, he didn't find the retreat nearly as physically challenging as I had. He took the vomiting in his stride: 'Mind over matter', he'd told me when I asked for a tip on coping with it. The few words he did express conveyed that he'd benefitted from all three ayahuasca experiences (and in a future email to me he'd write he was planning to do the retreat again).

I shared with the group what happened on my third trip, which seemed to leave everyone slightly blank, so I decided to ask a question that had been on my mind.

'Do you believe,' I looked at Carlos and Fanny, 'that whatever is happening is exactly what's supposed to be happening?'

'Yes, we do,' Fanny and Carlos said nodding together.

'I guess,' I suggested, 'what they say about trips, goes for daily life as well: you get the journey you need.'

'As I've been saying through the whole retreat,' Carlos responded gently, 'stop trying to control life. Whatever is happening can teach you something.'

It was the old Buddhist advice. Two words: let go.

'If I could bring myself to believe that everything that's happening is exactly what's supposed to be happening, it would reduce a lot of stress in my life. I found a simple Zen saying just before I left Australia that I think of often: "Obstacles do not block the path. They *are* the path".' Fanny and Carlos nodded in recognition.

I still couldn't imagine saying to a victim of crime, 'It was exactly what was supposed to happen! Just accept it.' Moreover, I'd spent my whole life saying, 'If you can't say it to an AIDS orphan in Africa, then it can't be true.' Why should a 'truth' apply for some middle-class white woman and not a victim of crime or an AIDS orphan?

It couldn't be denied, however, that my life would make more sense, there'd be less stress and I'd be happier if I could believe that everything that happened was supposed to happen. When people ask, would you rather be happy or right? I've usually chosen right. I guess I could run an experiment in my life of accepting 'everything is supposed to happen'. I can only live my own life, after all—and resign myself to the mystery of extreme suffering in the world and why it has to exist.

Soon after the retreat

It wouldn't be long before post-ayahuasca Sarah would be tested. I'd been exchanging a series of WhatsApp messages and emails with Pablo, the host of my next accommodation. I arrived with an uber driver, but I struggled to enter the flat as the door had an overwhelming arrangement of a lock box, a padlock and two keyholes. The driver stayed to help me and rang the landlord Pablo. I could hear Pablo on the speakerphone sounding annoyed. My Spanish kicked in when he said, '*Esta chica es completamente loca. Ella es de un otra planeta.*' In English: 'This woman is completely crazy. She's from another planet.' I interrupted their conversation to counter his claim: '*No soy loca y no soy de un otra planeta.*'

I eventually entered the apartment (Pablo had sent me the wrong code) and that night Pablo knocked on my window, which felt a little creepy. I opened the door, keeping the security door locked, and he apologised profusely for his behaviour earlier explaining that my call had occurred at a bad moment for him. I assumed he was only terrified I'd write a bad review and I responded without warmth.

The next day, in my wanders, my mind was consumed with the insult that I was crazy and from another planet and I even felt butterflies in my stomach as I tried to process this sudden threat to my clearly still-existent ego. I thought through all our communication by email and WhatsApp to ascertain why he would call me crazy. I nursed feelings of indignation and resentment towards this angry man. His poor wife, I tutted.

Before long, I caught myself: Haven't you taken anything away from that retreat? It's the same lesson you learned from the

Floridians: I am you and you are me. None of his behaviour was foreign to my own character. I too have been overwhelmed with stress. I've cursed people who got underfoot in the wrong moment. I've blamed others instead of owning my mood. These are not parts of myself that are easy to own, but I'm familiar with them. Pablo is me and I am Pablo and everyone is a potential spiritual teacher.

Weeks later

I continued to grapple with the 'Sarah Is Gone' moment in my second ayahuasca trip, mainly because I felt quite certain that she hadn't. After all, this moment had triggered my most dramatic vomit. Eventually, the experience would make more sense after reading the wise words of Dr Christopher Bache, who had taken LSD 73 times (and whose story appears in chapter 16 about LSD). In his book *LSD and the Mind of the Universe*, he wrote:

> What is the value of having visionary experiences in which one may touch a reality that is true but that one cannot keep on returning to ordinary consciousness?
>
> . . . The paradox is that something can be fully actualized in the psychedelic state and at the same time be incompletely realized inside the demanding conditions of space-time . . . It's all too easy to get carried away and think that more has been permanently accomplished in these hours than actually has been. But if we stay grounded in the reality of our incompleteness, a deeper dialectic begins to unfold.

> The birth of my Diamond Soul in session 38 gave me a foretaste of what I am in the process of becoming, and I believe this foretaste is helping me realize this destiny in my life. If held properly, these experiences begin to function as 'strange attractors,' pulling us toward our future through the increased awareness they bring. We may not be able to fully actualize these experiences immediately after a session has ended, but they bend the trajectory of our lives. In showing us what we are becoming, they help us become that very thing.[1]

I knew it would be important to revisit my 'Sarah Is Gone' ayahuasca memory as often as possible to remind myself of the direction I needed to head in.

Within two weeks of my arrival home, Luke and I broke up once and for all. As break ups go, it could only be described as acrimonious. While my preference is to 'consciously uncouple' and remain friends, this was not to be. We'd never speak again. That said, I mainly felt relief about my new freedom. It wasn't the first time I'd broken up with Luke as there'd been a blip in our compatibility even before my psychedelic journey had begun. On that occasion, after packing my bags and driving away, I'd panicked as I stared into an abyss of loneliness—only to fly back into his arms within hours.

Now I ask, who even *was* that woman? I'm a different person today—stronger, more positive, less vulnerable, happier, less anxious, more optimistic. I moved to the Sydney suburb of Newtown to the one-bedroom unit I'd bought and lived in during my late-twenties, back in the days when people in their twenties could afford real estate. I'd need to repaint and re-carpet and attend to the revolving door of tradesmen, but the effort of moving house, and setting up a new home, consumed my mental space.

Newtown has a buzz and it's loud. I need to wear noise-cancelling headphones most of the day and I'm three blocks back from King Street, the main street. Newtown thrums with curious visitors, a diversity of locals and youth that all look like art students. Bookshops, eateries and quirky shops stretch for miles. I adore the dog park and its adjoining cemetery, which boasts one of the best trees in Sydney, a Moreton Bay fig planted in 1848, at its entrance. To add to the welcome distractions, Alex and his girlfriend would join me, camping in the living room, for five weeks before they left for Europe to see Marek.

I continued to meditate daily as a way to keep all the realisations from ayahuasca alive. It was the best way to commune with the Divine Within, which I recognised more and more after every psychedelic experience. I'd soon find an integration therapist who also helped me to keep the realisations of my psychedelic journey alive.

Initially, I loved the single life and wondered how I ever could've worried about being lonely. Then again, I was busy, and living with my son and his girlfriend. When Alex left and the novelty of my new situation ended, things might be different.

16

Lead-up to LSD in Sydney

WHEN ALEX AND HIS girlfriend left, things were different. Realisations of just how alone I was hit me like a spray of bullets.

- I don't know a soul in Newtown.
- I face a string of empty weekends.
- I don't belong to any community.
- I have no colleagues.
- My friends live on the other side of the bridge and are absorbed with their own lives.

I couldn't even bury myself in work on the book as I was waiting for LSD to land in my letterbox, but that particular order never arrived (scammed!). My future seemed to stretch out in front of me bereft of company. I compulsively checked my phone all day, *Is anyone out there thinking of me?* but a watched pot never boils. I'd started to attend a Buddhist centre, and numerous classes at the gym, but knew it would take a long time to build connections. Moreover, at my age and given the three breakups of recent years,[1] my list of non-negotiables for any future partner was long.

An especially painful aspect of loneliness is the way you feel like you are the only one in a world of happily connected people. I, for one, am the only person among my friends who is unmarried let alone processing three relationship breakups in five years. All the books, however, emphasised that loneliness is universal, no one is spared. It's a part of every life, even for the happily married.

I'd had so much fun and laughter with both partners since my marriage split. The months of the honeymoon period, in each case, had been delightful, full of beaches, sunshine, bicycles, hikes, cocktails at lunch, the occasional long stint on a dance floor and deep sharing. Now, however, the pressure was on: I had to find the right man. If I chose the wrong person again, I'd be a card-carrying serial monogamist. Any more than three relationship breakdowns behind me might start to suggest it's *me* who's the problem. Still, I'd hold off until after the LSD in case it provided any insights on my situation.

Fortunately, the despair of loneliness would alternate with times when I relished the time alone—which was so confusing. During my past relationships I'd craved time by myself, even craved the breakup, yet could now see the potential to become way too isolated. On my worst day, I was teary all day before falling to the floor and sobbing, wishing my life was over, but knowing I could never inflict my demise on my sons. My future seemed bleak and

I became convinced this book would be a humiliating overshare with a depressing ending: Sarah abandoned.

I'm incredibly lucky that the deep depression only lasted two days. A harsh inner voice inquired, 'How can you sink so low after all the psychology you've studied, after the decades of Buddhist practice and meditation, after your whole psychedelic journey?' Thankfully, a kinder voice wondered, 'Maybe all those things contributed to the speed with which you were able to emerge from those depths?' I started to see that loneliness would come and go, just like any other internal weather. That said, by any objective measure, living alone at some distance from friends and family, I needed to actively seek out company.

Around this time, my Bufo-inspired six-month streak of living without sugar came to an abrupt halt as I started availing myself of Newtown's gourmet ice-creams, which were *soooo* comforting.

A return to the dating apps looked like the only answer but they were a threat to my mental health for so many reasons, not least, the inevitability of hurting the feelings of other lonely, vulnerable people. The first time I used dating apps was after my marriage ended, the boys had left home and I was home alone in the middle of a COVID lockdown. If I tried again now, the chances of finding someone on the same path as me, interested in spiritual growth and psychedelics, would be slim.

Fortunately, therapy was close at hand. Booked months ago, I had an appointment with a popular integration psychologist and my appointment was only a week away. Of course, I'd booked the appointment when I was on a post-ayahuasca high and now that I felt less buoyant, I wished I'd chosen a therapist of my own gender and around my age.

Loneliness

In the meantime, I did what I always do when despair knocks at my door and buried myself in books to research my predicament. Reading about other people's loneliness comforted me in mine. In the book *Alone,* which I sometimes hold against my heart, German author Daniel Schreiber suffered painful loneliness as a single man during a COVID lockdown. He wrote that to speak of our loneliness feels like a social taboo: 'the lonelier I felt the less I could talk about it. And the less I talked about it the lonelier I felt.'[2] He'd believed himself deserted by friends during COVID but worked through his feelings: '. . . I had disregarded perhaps the only basic rule of friendship: that friendships are based on freedom, not on social constraints or institutionalized obligations. Friends do not have to conform to one's own wishes, expectations and demands.'

In *Solitude and Loneliness*, English Buddhist Sarvananda writes, 'A clear-sighted acknowledgement of our essential aloneness is where the spiritual life begins.'[3] He quotes the Buddha, 'Be islands unto yourselves, refuges unto yourselves, seeking no external refuge.' To benefit from a spiritual life, Sarvananda argues, we need to foster a capacity to be alone and self-sufficient, rather than to endlessly distract ourselves, or seek the company of others as soon as we feel the slightest twinge of loneliness. Yet, Sarvananda also emphasised, as did the Buddha, the importance of spiritual community. I knew, however, that I needed deeper connections than I could find attending Tuesday meditation group. Sometimes, if I'd prioritised finding new friends, or a potential partner, I'd return home after a meditation evening feeling even more sad—making strong connections in a new community takes time and it's easy to question whether it'll ever happen.

Fun facts about LSD

Getting back down to work on my book, I'd planned a background chapter on LSD only to find that most of my points were covered in the first episode of Michael Pollan's Netflix series *How To Change Your Mind*. Some months back, when I'd watched the series, I'd started on the second episode about psilocybin, which had been more my focus at the time.[4] Pollan narrated how: LSD is not addictive; there's no known lethal dose; and, between 1950 and 1965 a thousand scientific articles about it were written based on 40,000 research subjects.

My favourite quotation, from the same episode, was from Jim Fadiman, the 'Father of Microdosing', when he said: 'I took LSD and that was the day my life was transformed. Where I realized that Jim Fadiman, for all of his benefits and flaws, was a subset of a larger being and that larger being was connected to all other beings.' Later in the episode, Fadiman describes an experiment he ran where *all* of 48 scientists who took an LSD trip found 'satisfactory solutions' to questions they'd been stuck on for over three months.

Such results make it less surprising that two Nobel prizewinners—biochemist Kary Mullis and molecular biologist Francis Crick—had a history of taking LSD to promote creative thinking. Mullis gives significant credit for his breakthrough to the 'mind-opening experiences' provided by LSD: 'What if I had not taken

LSD ever; would I have still invented PCR [polymerase chain reaction]? I don't know. I doubt it. I seriously doubt it.'[5]

Taking LSD 73 times

One seasoned explorer of LSD is an emeritus professor who taught philosophy and religious studies for 33 years and twice won his university's Distinguished Professor award. Inspired by the writings of Stanislav Grof, Dr Christopher Bache embarked on his own necessarily secret project, which would see him take a high dose of LSD 73 times over twenty years in therapeutically structured sessions. In the introduction to his book *LSD and the Mind of the Universe*, he writes:

> I hope the fact that I have lived a socially responsible and engaged life will give me a small measure of credibility when I tell the unusual story that follows.[6]

Dr Bache writes that he was not seeking healing so much as an understanding of the universe. He believes he pushed himself way too hard with dosages from 500–600 micrograms when the 'therapeutic' dose some experts recommend is 50–200. He'd advise others to be gentler on themselves but claims that those 73 days were the most important of his life. One of the hardest aspects of his LSD odyssey was the loneliness. With the war on drugs, he wouldn't be able to share his discoveries with his colleagues, students and friends, and this was painfully isolating.

I read his book a full year ago but many moments have lingered in my mind. His first 'ego death', for example, forced him 'to become the exact opposite of everything I had ever known myself to be . . . I was being stripped of my maleness and trapped in the lives of women'. Another memorable point was his firm belief in reincarnation, which 'wove itself in and out of my sessions many times'.[7] He subscribes to a theory that before our birth 'we consciously choose our next life on earth' from among several possibilities, based on 'the opportunities each offers us to grow and develop'. It struck me that embracing this concept, if I could, had the potential to reframe life's difficulties as important opportunities for learning that might benefit me not just in this life, but for future incarnations as well.

Most memorably of all, Dr Bache saw the future of humanity. His journeys showed him that humanity will endure a time of terrible suffering triggered by ecological crises. Our collective pain will become so unbearable that it will force us to make changes that will lead to the emergence of a new form of human, a Future Human.

> The ecological crisis will precipitate a death-rebirth confrontation that will shatter our psycho-spiritual isolation, both individually and societally, and bring forward an awakening of common ground within us. We will look with amazement at the depth of ignorance that had set us on this course of self-decimation, and we will not long for that past at all . . . What a magnificent being! Just touching it filled me with rapture, calm, and sheer delight. It felt clear, warm, and whole. There was an abiding sense of Oneness that went deeper than just the

feeling of being interconnected. It was a feeling of being truly One underneath the diversity of life.

Needless to say, each Future Human would be the culmination of numerous incarnations over time. The Future Human might include the souls of you and me, once we've learned all our lessons.

First preparation meeting with Dr Max

The challenge with LSD would be to create that all-important safe container. While I was able to take psilocybin, Bufo and ayahuasca in a shamanic container, LSD had been discovered by a Swiss chemist, so I was aware of no rituals or traditions around its use other than the dubious container of 'sixties culture' or more recently 'recreational drug taking'. Nor did MDMA come with ancient rituals, but my qualified underground psychotherapist, Sasha, had provided a therapeutic setting complete with a trip-sitting service.

With LSD I'd be left to my own devices. I'd need to create my own set and setting and wanted to do it safely, responsibly and in a way that showed respect for the medicine. I found an integration psychologist online with impressive credentials. I'd make several face-to-face appointments with Dr Max and commit to the therapy. Dr Max, to my surprise, would offer a way for LSD to happen in both a therapeutic *and* a spiritual container.

Meeting Dr Max in person was confirmation that he was considerably younger than me, yet once we started talking it was clear he had the empathy, intelligence and maturity for the job. I told him about my past trips and what I'd learned from them, especially about my new relationship with the crying baby, needy toddler and depressed adult of ten years ago. I provided the short version of my life story and where I was at in my life, including that now I felt very alone and didn't know what to do about it.

'I'm actually feeling quite defeatist,' I admitted. 'I know that I'll never have the thing I want more than anything, a sense of belonging to a group, or even a partner who cares for me. I'm just not a charismatic person, I'm not a people magnet.'

Even I was surprised, though, at the thing that made me burst into tears. It sounded childish, but there it was: 'If I could have one thing, more than anything in the world, I'd love it if someone organised a surprise party for me—I know it's dumb—but the point is that it could never, ever happen. The friends I have left barely even know each other anyway.'

'It's not dumb at all,' said Dr Max. 'You just want to feel that others are thinking about you in a kind way. It's perfectly normal.'

We were running out of time, but Dr Max wrapped it up saying: 'Sarah, I know you feel defeatist, but with therapy you can heal. You'll uncover times from your past that will break your heart, but I assure you that you can heal. That's why you're on this psychedelic journey, this spiritual journey.'

For two seconds I felt hope that he was right and therapy might be the answer, but I also wondered if his words were just marketing to ensure I booked more appointments.

Second meeting with Dr Max

'So how did you feel after last week?' Dr Max asked.

'I actually felt very depressed for the rest of the day and well into the next day, but I managed to climb out of the hole with some self-care and I feel fine now.'

Dr Max nodded knowingly. 'Why do you think you felt so down?'

'I guess last week's session stirred up thoughts and memories that I suppress so I can get on with life.'

'Therapy's definitely a messy business because parts of you feel threatened by it, by the prospect of change, so they act out or mount resistance. Have you heard of Internal Family Systems therapy?' he asked.

'I have a vague feeling that's what Sasha, the MDMA therapist, used when we talked about my inner crying baby and tantrumming toddler.'

'It's based on the work of a Dr Schwartz who came to the conclusion, after years of working with his patients, that none of us are monolithic entities but that we're each made up of a multiplicity of parts. No matter how any of these parts behave, there are no bad parts, as the purpose of every one of them is to protect you.'

'So we work to get rid of the unhelpful ones?' I asked.

'That's where people go astray. Every part, no matter how extreme, has your best interests at heart—they want to protect you from what they think you can't handle or what might overwhelm you—so we aren't trying to squash or kill any.'

'Okay, I think I'm probably guilty of trying to squash or kill parts,' I speculated.

'Instead, therapy is about listening to each part and what they have to say. The focus is on releasing what Schwartz calls the "burdens" of our parts, not the parts themselves. If the parts feel heard and understood, they may gradually quieten down or feel ready for a new more helpful role. All parts need to feel welcome just like each member of a family, no matter how obnoxious, needs to feel valued in order for the system to work at its best.'

'Does that mean your job as the therapist is to identify the parts, listen to them and negotiate?'

'No, actually. I can facilitate the process and may occasionally detect a part that you have overlooked, but there's something inside each one of us that Schwartz calls the "Self"—capital S—who does the work, both within and outside therapy, and long after therapy is over. Only the Self knows how to heal the parts and the speed of healing that your system can cope with. The Self is far more knowledgeable about your needs than I can be.'

'Wow, this sounds like psychology meets spirituality.'

'Most people do see it that way. The Self—capital S—could also go by the name of Buddha Nature or the seat of consciousness, the Higher Self or even the Divine or the Beloved, depending on your spiritual background.'

This was the moment I realised we could create a container for psychedelic experiences that was both therapeutic and spiritual.

'Ayahuasca gave me the message that the Divine is inside me, even maybe the Holy Spirit,' I said with air-quotes for the Holy Spirit.

'It so happens,' replied Dr Max, 'that the Self is naturally compassionate and kind to you, and to everyone else, so all the parts can learn to trust the Self.'

'That resembles another insight I had doing ayahuasca. A bird landed on the shoulder of the Sarah who lay in her bed depressed, ten years ago, and inquired, "Why couldn't you be there for yourself?". It was reminding me that the Self can be there if I let it, with compassion and kindness, for any part when it suffers.'

'Exactly,' said Dr Max. 'The Self knows how to heal us, emotionally, and work with the innate capacity of our bodies and minds for healing. The goal is to gradually transition to being Self-led instead of allowing our various parts to run the show.'

'Self-led,' I repeated, to lock it into my mind. 'I'm sure meditation is a great way to be more in touch with that Self so that it can be more available to work with all the different parts?'

'Meditation is especially helpful for this,' Dr Max agreed. I remembered the first time I'd ever spoken to Dr Max on the phone, he'd apologised for taking a while to get back to me as he'd been on a meditation retreat.

'It's also important to understand,' Dr Max continued, 'that parts are not just random voices in your head, or even emotional states like "sadness" or "anger", but fully fledged sub-personalities who have a story and a wide range of beliefs and emotions. They're inner characters that stopped developing at a certain age in response to trauma or distressing events. Parts often disagree with each other, creating what Schwartz called polarisations, so a lot of therapy is about understanding these inner conflicts.'

I would later read that all parts are 'protectors' and fall into three categories: managers, exiles and firefighters. Managers tend to bully or suppress the 'weak, vulnerable' exiled parts whereas the firefighters want to help the exiles feel less pain. Firefighters offer solutions that distract, numb or anaesthetise us—alcohol, overeating, porn or even endless hours of television can be behaviours that firefighters use to help us muffle the moans of our exiled parts. Managers and firefighters are often at cross-purposes. Yet the longer the exiles are suppressed, or anaesthetised, the more extreme they grow.[8]

I couldn't believe how I'd missed the opportunity to learn about this therapy from Sasha, my MDMA therapist, as I'd been avoiding therapy back then; not to mention that I'd used my time with her to make sense of my ailing relationship with Luke.

What does Internal Family Systems therapy have to do with psychedelics?

I quickly became smitten with Internal Family Systems therapy (IFS) and how it combined the therapeutic and the spiritual. In my excitement, I bought all Dr Schwartz's books about it.

Dr Richard C. Schwartz was well-versed in the latest research on MDMA for treating depression. In his book for practitioners, *Internal Family Systems Therapy*, he alludes to the MDMA research by IFS therapists Dr Michael Mithoefer, and his wife Annie, who noticed in their MDMA sessions with study participants that 'the vast majority of participants began to speak about and interact with their parts' without any prior direction from the therapists. In one of their studies of PTSD sufferers, 92 per cent of them reported 'greater understanding and acceptance of these parts'. Interviewed by Dr Schwarz, Dr Mithoefer stated that MDMA allowed participants to skip many steps in the usual process of IFS therapy so that clients could 'move quickly into witnessing and unburdening exiles'.[9]

Dr Schwartz elaborates:

> I have watched videos of several sessions conducted by Michael and Annie Mithoefer, both IFS therapists, which illustrate the subjects accessing an enormous amount of Self with great speed, and parts healing spontaneously. Their magnified access to the Self seems to reassure and convert protectors quickly.

Ironically, I was learning about many of my parts around the time of taking LSD, rather than MDMA, although MDMA had undeniably done the heavy lifting after revealing my inner baby and toddler parts. The process of uncovering parts had been under way before I understood it. I wondered if the involuntary moans that had lasted four days after I took MDMA, were the moans of a long-suppressed exile within.

Preparation for LSD with Dr Max

After discussing Parts Therapy—another name for Internal Family Systems therapy—Dr Max and I discussed my plan of taking the LSD as part of a small group at the home of a new psychedelic-interested friend in a different city.

'My focus is always on safety,' Dr Max began, 'not just physical safety but emotional safety. When you take it with people you know there are always friendship dynamics. I have to say I can see some red flags in your plan.'

I could see them too now. 'I walk on eggshells as a guest in someone's home and if my trip is long I might feel like I'm outstaying my welcome. Even more important, if the LSD makes me act weirdly, I wouldn't want to be with people I don't know very well.'

'Well, do listen to those concerns,' advised Dr Max. 'Explore them. They sound like things that may get in the way of your ability to truly let go to the experience.'

'You're probably right. I'm also worried about driving home afterwards, or even being on a train. What if it takes a while for me to recover?'

'I don't want to tell you what to do,' said Dr Max, 'only that you need to take the time to listen to what some of your parts have to say about this plan, because if you silence them, they may demand to be heard during the trip. Explore your options until you feel your parts say, "that makes sense".'

Dr Max had helped me to put myself first to design a scenario that met my needs. He helped me listen to the 'still, quiet voice within', which I too easily ignore. I decided to abandon the group-setting idea and take the LSD in my own home. My friend Trish and I would trip on separate days so that we could be present for each other as trip-sitters.

'Do you have any concerns about your friend Trish?' Dr Max asked.

'Not Trish, per se. My only concern is the social need to chat in the lead-up and chatting takes me up into my head. One of the insights from ayahuasca was to rely less on language, words and concepts, so I'd rather begin the trip from a place of stillness, from a meditative place. My mind is chatty enough on its own without chatting out loud with someone.'

We decided that Trish would arrive at my home a few minutes before I take the LSD so there'd be no chatting time. Before the day, I'd have a conversation with her about my desire to avoid conversation.

I took Dr Max's parting words to me as a compliment: 'I'd say you're equipped, Sarah, with the most important quality you need for your trip and that's curiosity.'

Trish

I'd met Trish at university in my early twenties. I knew she'd be up for trying LSD as she'd always been adventurous, fun and open to new experiences. She had a little background in recreational drug-taking from her youth but, true to character, was open to a novel approach where we'd prioritise personal growth—and safety.

Trish had, in fact, tried LSD before and recounted: 'My friend Louise and I took it decades ago and we were happily painting a wall in our house, when our friend Sebastian turned up out of the blue.' I decided not to inquire why she would be painting a wall while tripping on acid. 'He bundled us into his car, drove us to the middle of nowhere and left us there to somehow make our way home. That was Sebastian's idea of a hilarious prank. It was pretty stressful in the state we were in. I had bad stomach cramps from the LSD as well.' She was still keen to give LSD another try in a better setting.

Trish had enjoyed some fun experiences with psychedelics too, such as when, aged twenty, she took psilocybin with friends on a holiday in Byron Bay where she remembers regally striding through the streets accompanied, she believed, by 50 white horses.

She took mushrooms on another occasion, with her friend Helen, in the town of Nimbin. She remembers seeing the 'life energy, in the form of tiny diamonds, travelling through the plants'. She was an art student at the time and the visuals had been so stunning that they inspired her next year of work for college. Eventually, Helen and Trish entered a pub where Trish swears she saw the actor Matthew McConaughey when he came to Australia in his youth, well before his fame. She stood in front of him, gazing into his eyes and declared, 'You're the most beautiful man I've ever seen.'

'Why, thank you,' replied Matthew in his Southern drawl, at which point Helen grabbed Trish's arm and dragged her out to continue wandering. Trish finished her trip in a field engaged in a long talk to a real horse.

'How sure are you that it was Matthew McConaughey?' I asked Trish, decades later.

She paused to think before answering with deadpan expression: 'Ninety-eight per cent'.

17

LSD in Sydney

Almost a year ago now, before I attended the psilocybin retreat, a caring friend had phoned me.

'Remind me, which drug are you taking in the Netherlands?'

'Psilocybin,' I replied. 'Y'know, magic mushrooms.'

'Oh phew, for a moment I thought you'd be taking LSD.'

Hahaha, we chuckled. I didn't bother telling her that I had every intention of taking LSD and was looking forward to it.

After a couple of frustrating false starts I managed to source some. At first, I thought I'd received an empty envelope but a closer look revealed the ten tabs, which together, looked the size of a postage stamp, each tab, or square, measuring six-by-six millimetres. My information, for what it's worth, was that it was a form of LSD called Needlepoint, apparently the purest form. I followed my testing-kit instructions and, over a white plate, cut a corner, the size of a bread crumb, off one of the tabs. I'd drop a drip of testing liquid on the sample and if LSD was present, the speck would turn purple. The instructions said, 'The reaction can take several minutes, so be patient.' I released the drop and watched the speck instantly turn purple. My new favourite colour.

The night before, some lower back pain came to a head and I couldn't find a comfortable position. I hoped the LSD would fix it. I'd ask it.

Knowing I could be tripping for twelve hours, I'd organised for my son Zac to come over after his work at around 7 p.m. to relieve Trish. As it happened, Zac had taken a small dose of psilocybin with friends the previous weekend so there'd be plenty to talk about.

First LSD trip

Trish arrived at 8.50 a.m. and we set her up with my Wi-Fi password and a workstation, so she could do her own thing as she trip-sat me. After all, I couldn't expect her to meditate, or watch me, for the many hours ahead. My phone pinged with a message from Dr Max:

> Hi Sarah, just wanted to offer you a quote: 'Healing is not becoming the best version of yourself. Healing is letting the worst version of yourself be loved.'

His message would influence my very first vision on the trip.

I chewed up one tiny tab plus a little extra, which came to 130 micrograms, and inserted my ear buds to access my playlist. Lying on the couch, I had no fear but, as is my pattern, worried that nothing would happen—the tab was so small, how could it have any power? Yet within what felt like ten minutes, my head was shaking back and forth and the trembling throughout my body grew fierce.

Please fix my back! I start with a request.

I'm a giant pelican princess—in technicolour—with the longest of legs attended by two equally lofty pelican nurses. They remove a large colourful rock from my chest, which feels like the removal of emotional pain that has collected there. The nurses marvel at the colours in the rock and assure me that the rock is precious.

The scene changes: a take-charge-type caveman arrives in a room that symbolises my mind. He looks around to survey how best to clean up this place and rubs his hands together to start work . . .

I begin sobbing hard and know I'm releasing the pain of loneliness, feeling that I cry for the loneliness of all humanity.

I've completely left my current life behind. I know this feeling from past trips and feel bemused again that I ever assumed life on earth was the only reality. I'm aware that Trish is asking if I'm okay and I laugh at her—the poor thing thinks she's in reality. The flow of images is fast-moving and hectic—sometimes I move through a swampy forest, other times I sit in a meeting room at the top of a skyscraper trying to nail down the meaning of life in discussions with those in power: 'So we know you can't work it out through intelligence. We can rule that out.' We are so close to getting it but there's always an outstanding question we can't answer.

Multiple images appear—smiling female zombies, intricate tree root systems that morph into the veins in the zombie's bodies, skulls, plump cavemen. Through all the signs and symbols I reach a realisation: every human being is a manifestation of me—we're all the same thing. The men, women and children, they are all my parts.

But who is me? I don't know who I am anymore. I've forgotten. What gender am I? I'm on a quest to arrive back at me but it takes a journey through rainy forests. I enjoy the mission. I keep calling Zac's name, which seems like the key to making it back. I hear Trish say, 'He's coming later'.

Finally, I arrive back in the room and feel disoriented. My body feels puffy and bloated, my vision is blurry. I look at my watch and wonder if it's upside down. Or maybe on the wrong wrist. I can't read the time for a while but when I can I understand it's been seven hours. I'm aware that I've survived the peak and lie a little longer in my heavy body.

I'm full of wonder and awe at what just happened but notice that I don't feel the usual euphoria. In fact, I feel irritable. My ear buds have fallen out exposing me to the noise that comes from living in Newtown—the passing cars, people in the street, the neighbour's television. I feel hypersensitive to noise and it's making me cranky. I see Trish at her computer and feel disconnected from her. This is the wrong setting! I should be in nature, with people sharing the experience.

It's grey and drizzly outside and I feel claustrophobic. Even the fact that it's a Tuesday makes me feel isolated—who does acid on a cloudy, wet Tuesday, for God's sake? I feel lonely and desolate; rather than learning how to cope with my aloneness, I only feel more determined to find my person who could be there for me on future trips.

I sit up but my body feels weighted down and I'm dizzy. A little chatter with Trish cheers me up and we decide to go for a walk.

Sitting on the grass in the park, I enthuse to Trish about my trip but then complain about the setting, and we chat about how she might approach her turn.

'Lots of people in the psychedelic world,' I said, 'talk about what the best container or cultural context might be for Westerners taking the medicines in the future. People with mental illness will use a clinical setting, but what about the rest of us? We can't suddenly transplant shamanism into the West.'

'My experiences from my twenties,' said Trish, 'have been in the outdoors in company, but a problem can be when another person's experience affects yours, like if they start bossing you around and expect you to play a role in their psychodrama.'

'I haven't had an experience on psychedelics of wandering around with my eyes open and interacting with others. I'd probably need a low dose as I usually feel too heavy to be upright.'

'I've found that I just want to go and *play* and explore the new worlds before me.'

I had an idea: 'Maybe in the future when the laws loosen up, we should have like children's play centres for adults. So they can take their psychedelic medicine and then be let loose to play in sandpits, Lego pits, with Play-Doh and dress-up boxes. And you could have sober "parent figures" to supervise. That way parents could be parented while they play—they'd love that!'

Oh dear. The ideas you come up with when on acid. I'd only forgotten to say 'Man!'

Back at my unit, I bade Trish goodbye and lay my heavy body down for a couple of hours before Zac arrived. I didn't enjoy the way my body felt, like it had a flu, and it reminded me of that first time I took psilocybin back in the living room of the family home.

Later, I defrosted a chicken curry and chatted with Zac.

'We just had a low dose,' said Zac. 'I'm done with high doses for the time being.'

'So it was you and your girlfriend, your best friend and another friend,' I confirmed, 'and you were on the beach.'

'Yeah. We just had fun and enjoyed each other's company.'

'Wow, Zac. I'm so jealous. That's the setting I crave. A trip-sitter to keep a watch on everyone would make it ideal, though.'

I felt a momentary sadness. It was hard enough to find a partner, let alone a partner I could trip with, not to mention a small group of friends open to psychedelics.

The sadness quickly dissipated, though, as there is no greater joy than chatting about the medicines with your adult children. It opens up so many topics—psychology, spirituality, personal histories. It's a rich topic for discussion and it gives me a chance to remind them about safety considerations.

The next day, although I needed paracetamol for my headache and a few lie-downs for the lingering exhaustion, I was thrilled to confirm my back pain had gone. I would still have my usual stiff lower back but the intense pain of the night before, which had built up over the previous week, had disappeared. In recent years, sitting for any amount of time had triggered lower back pain. Psychedelics had relieved this for me, but only for a day or two. My lower back pain would eventually disappear further down the track, after I followed my son Zac's advice, 'You just need to strengthen your glutes'. He was right—it worked and only after a couple of weeks of exercises. Psychedelics, apparently work best on the pain caused by stored emotions that we haven't resolved.

A shoulder ache had also gone. For weeks, I hadn't been able to do a single push-up and the exercises a physio once suggested when my shoulder flared up years ago hadn't helped, but today I could do push-ups completely free of pain. Admittedly, the shoulder pain would return in about three weeks but I appreciated the break.

On the previous weekend, the topic of psychedelics for pain had been on my radar, as I'd been at a picnic with a group I'd met online who hold gatherings to chat about plant medicines. I'd been to a few such events with various groups, underground and above ground, and I sometimes met people who suffered from chronic physical pain that made their life miserable. I met three such people at the picnic, who all happened to be parents of young children.

Two of them had tried other forms of pain relief but knew that a psychedelic medicine—psilocybin for one of them, LSD for the other—was all that worked for them. The third wanted to try psilocybin for the first time as nothing had helped her in the past. She'd suffered financial loss when she tried to purchase some psilocybin 'chocolate bars' online, only to be scammed. When I met her, she'd braved Sydney Sunday traffic to attend the picnic, where she feverishly networked to find someone who might help her. I exchanged some texts with her a few weeks later, after she'd managed to source, and try, microdosing[1] psilocybin:

> I am very pleased with how it's going. Psilocybin has definitely helped me, it has been the best thing that's happened to me in a long time!

Unconscionable is one word to describe the situation where a suffering person finally finds a solution to long-term pain but has no way to access that solution legally. Of course, it's the same situation for plenty of people with treatment-resistant depression and PTSD who struggle to access what can heal them. Not that psychedelics will necessarily cure everyone but suffering people should, at least, be able to explore the options, just in case.

Trish's turn

Trish also chose to take her LSD trip in the safety of her own home and chose a day when the rest of her family members were away. I was excited about my first trip-sitting gig and complied with Trish's request to arrive early in the morning.

'Have you thought about an intention?' I asked Trish as we sat at her breakfast table.

'Yes, I feel that after all the struggles of family life, and trying to make my career work, I want to let go more. I go through life like a tight fist and I'd like to be more loosened up.'

'Okay, good one. Dosage?'

'No idea, what do you think?'

'Depends whether you want to play it safe and treat today as dipping-your-toe-in-the-water, or if you want something stronger. There's no known lethal dose.'

'How much did you have?'

'I only had 130 micrograms and managed to visit another dreamlike world but I'm small and sensitive.'

'I'll try 150.'

I cut her a square and a half with my Stanley knife, which she drank down with water. I soon worried that the water may have diluted it but left her to meditate in her living room while I set up in her back courtyard.

Trish's experience, using the same batch of LSD, seemed completely different to mine.

For starters, she claimed after an hour that she couldn't feel anything whereas I'd turned into a pelican princess after twenty minutes on a smaller dose. After some googling of one of the many psychedelic discussion forums, we decided that she should take another half tab and let it dissolve under her tongue. About twenty minutes later, she smiled broadly. 'It's working now.'

Over the next few hours, Trish only spent around an hour lying down whereas I'd had no choice but to lie my heavy body down for hours. Trish drew pictures of the geometric patterns she saw, she danced, she wandered around her house, she cried a lot, she laughed.

She spent time thinking through problematic relationships and seeing them through a different lens. She found more compassion for the main characters in her life and also for herself. Trish had an 'eyes open' experience, which I was yet to have. She marvelled at how every object pulsated, throbbed or swayed. Best of all, every object had a rainbow aura. We spent a couple of hours chatting after the peak and I observed that she could barely stop laughing even though the topics she spoke of were all quite serious. I must've looked confused by this dissonance but she didn't seem to notice. Was this behaviour evidence that she'd fulfilled her intention of letting go and taking things less seriously?

It turned out that Trish had seen visions that gave her a chance to observe all her 'efforting' over the years and she saw that so much of it felt absurd and unnecessary. Why not perform the same actions with a light touch rather than the tight fist? She found herself laughing at how hard she'd always tried. While watching these visions of herself throughout her life, she realised, *I've done a lot. I've seen a lot. I'm a mature person now, so I'm strong.* Although she believed she'd had a 'strong dose', she didn't experience any particular body sensations, nothing mystical, no visits to other dimensions. Still, she seemed delighted with her experience and found it 'so interesting' and 'really fun'.

Within 24 hours of her trip, Trish made a difficult phone call she'd been putting off and marvelled at how strong she felt and how assertive she could be. When I spoke to her, she seemed proud of how she dealt with the call, 'I feel like I'd witnessed myself in a new way during the trip and I want to hang onto the more authentic me I uncovered'.

A few weeks later I spoke to Trish again about the effects of her trip.

'I feel so much more love and appreciation for my husband,' she enthused. This warmed my heart as I have a high opinion of her husband, a man of great depth with a huge social conscience. She also spoke of some more difficult conversations that had tested her and credited her LSD trip for her strengthened confidence to express her point of view.

Integration with Dr Max

I read my trip report out to Dr Max.

'Tell me what you'd like to focus on,' he asked. 'What resonates most for you?'

'Maybe the insight that every human I meet is just a part of me. We're all the same stuff, although I have to say, it felt so clear in the trip. Now, in the clear light of day, I find it a lot to get my head around.'

'Why do you think that feels important for you?'

'It builds on what I learned from the ayahuasca retreat.' I told Dr Max about the two Floridians and how I grew so fond of two people who were different to me and how I saw them as manifestations of parts of myself, even though I didn't know about parts therapy back then.

'Is there a way that you can apply this in your daily life, this idea that every human is a part of you?'

'It can help me to cope with difficult people, or people who I perceive as different to me. I think I'm naturally quite judgemental and intolerant, whereas I want to be compassionate and loving.'

'I can see a duality there, Sarah. You have a part that you call judgemental and intolerant, and then another part that wants to be compassionate and loving that disapproves of the judgemental part.'

'But isn't the part that wants to be compassionate and loving the Self? We're not talking about two polarised parts, are we?'

'We are if there's a *should* involved and I'm hearing a part that says, *I should be compassionate and loving.* With the Self there are no *shoulds.* The Self never has an agenda.'

'Right,' I realise. 'The Self is naturally compassionate and loving. There's no big stick.'

'And remember the part you see as intolerant and judgemental is only trying to protect you, like any part. It exists for a reason.'

'I can see the tendency of the part that says "should" to try to clobber the parts of me that don't conform to a Buddhist ideal.'

'Yes, but all parts need to feel heard, understood and loved. One of my favourite quotes is: "If you want to let go, you must fall in love with the part of you that's holding on".'[2]

'That's beautiful.' I write it down and continue, 'I can see that the part of me that says "should" tries to drown some of my parts, or bash them with a baseball bat, but that reaction to my own parts means I'll be judgemental and intolerant of those around me who display equivalent parts.'

'We can't authentically love others,' said Dr Max, 'until we love all the parts of ourselves, without exception. I have a feeling there are other moments in your life when this "should" part beats you up.'

'I can think of one now,' I answered. 'I know I can feel triggered, or irritated when I feel someone has said something dumb, or ignorant, but then I feel incredibly disappointed with myself for feeling irritated because I'm not being nice. I suspect my irritable part is only reacting to my anxiety about whether I'm intelligent myself so I can't stand seeing a lack of intelligence in others that reminds me of that anxiety.'

Dr Max summarised, 'So we have a part that's irritated because it's worried about your own intelligence and a part saying you shouldn't feel irritated with others. Can you see the polarisation?'

I nodded.

'That hang-up about intelligence,' Dr Max continued, 'came up during the LSD trip: in those boardrooms where you tried to nail down the meaning of life. I remember you said the discussions started from the base that intelligence won't bring you any closer to the answers.'

'I guess the message there,' I offered, 'from that feeling of never quite getting the meaning of life, is that it's unknowable. It's a mystery and that's the way it's going to stay. You can't think, study or read your way to an answer. All you can do is try to live in the present and be kind to yourself and others.'

'Are you sure,' asked Dr Max, 'you can't think of one other interpretation of the meaning of life based on your psychedelic journey to date?'

'I guess a lot of psychonauts and spiritual types find from their trips that the meaning of life is "love". You don't need intelligence to understand that. The message from my first ayahuasca trip ties in here: don't rely on language and words or intelligence. Live from your heart. Stop hiding up in your head.'

'So the meaning of life is to love but I think you've discovered one other thing that it might be about. Let's go back to you as the pelican princess and how a colourful rock of your pain was removed and found to be precious. What do you make of that?'

'I think it ties back to the quote you texted me: *Healing is letting the worst version of yourself be loved*. It's about admitting there's value in the painful parts of yourself.'

'And what is the value of pain, for you?'

'Well, I guess you learn valuable lessons when you suffer—it's a golden opportunity to work with your exiled parts, as you call them, to get to know them better, and give them some love. They won't reveal themselves unless we go through some pain.'

'Yep,' affirmed Dr Max, 'they all have your best interests at heart, they're all trying to protect you. They just might not understand the best way to do that because many of them are very young, children even. But it's inspiring that if we unburden our parts, we can give them new jobs such as reminding us to see the humour, or to be playful or even to forgive others.'

'I've just remembered now, in my Bufo journey, that message I saw in capitals: PAIN IS MY TEACHER. That ties in too. To be honest, I'd rather do my learning from a nice self-help book, but there's nothing like lived experience, I suppose.'

'Our parts are definitely teachers,' replied Dr Max, 'if we make the space to listen to them.'

It was dawning on me that the meaning of life was love but also learning. Personal growth, or learning. Those who believe in reincarnation say that we keep returning to relive more lives until we've learned all our lessons and finally 'awaken' into who we are supposed to be.

The message was coming from several directions: I needed to reframe the difficulties in life to see them as valuable teachers. Again, that Zen quote: 'Obstacles do not block the path; they are the path.'

18

Second LSD trip in Sydney

For my second LSD trip I was determined to improve on the setting. My son Alex had returned from Europe to live with me in Newtown until he found a place, and he agreed to gift me his Friday to trip-sit me. This time, I wanted an outdoor setting in nature, with privacy. I decided on the back lawn of my mother's house where she'd lived for almost 60 years, my childhood home.

When Friday arrived, I was keen to leave Newtown for my mother's house early but Alex was still jetlagged and had slept in. I knew he had plans for the evening and I was growing irritable, not with Alex, but with the situation. He clearly wouldn't be able to give me the twelve hours I might need. When we eventually got on the road, I realised that I hadn't settled on an intention. I decided on, 'To address my irritability and impatience'. Like many women, socialised to be nice, I rarely inflicted my irritability on others, but I was aware of the 'grumpy old woman' that could percolate under the surface on a bad day.

On my first LSD trip, a week and a half ago, I'd ingested 130 micrograms, on a cloudy day in noisy Newtown. On today's trip I'd take 170 micrograms, on a warm, sunny day, in a peaceful suburb in Sydney's leafy north. This time only a thin mattress would separate me from the earth. My shaded spot on the lawn overlooked a verdant valley, full of bird life, trees swaying in the breeze—a view dotted with the mauve of jacaranda flowers. I set up under the shade of a tree and Alex would lie metres away, in a tent, reading a book.

No trip report

The trip was intense but I couldn't write about it as there was almost a complete lack of narrative and it's hard to remember details. Again, I travelled through time to another era and was conscious that my body, shuddering as usual, received a thorough workout. It felt like every cell enjoyed a cleanout and I could feel swirls of stale energy departing my skin from all over my body.

Some of the themes were the same as my first LSD trip: what is the meaning of life and who's running the show? Visions of my sons; amnesia about who I was; and again, the quest to make my way back through time to return to my spot in the universe.

I also revisited the theme of 'I am you'. This time I spent a fair while occupying the body of a plump teenage boy as he wandered around a shopping mall in Texas looking for donuts. Yep, I'm him. I'm anyone. I'm everyone. They're all me. I'm all of them.

I'd asked Alex to take notes if I said anything and this is what he recorded me saying a few hours in:

> So many places to get back through to get back to here . . .
> There are portals to the spirit world, all the time, everywhere.
> Somebody has got to be responsible for everything. Who's running this ecosystem? Whose vision is all this? I don't understand who's in charge?
> I'm just with my grandma now.
> I need to get plugged back into the system. How do I start to find my way back?

In the minutes before I landed back in my body, I had a vision of a puddle of paint spilt on the road.

> Something the size and shape of a chicken's egg was lying in the paint. On closer inspection it turned out to be the head of a tired, wizened little old lady in the form of a Leunig character—bulbous nose and a scowl—but she was adorable and I realised she was my grumpy old lady part, otherwise known as my irritable part.

What a slow learner I'd been when I'd made the intention to 'address' my irritability. Once again, I'd sought to murder a part of myself instead of making the space to listen to and love it. I scooped the grumpy old lady up and put her in an imaginary pocket, thinking to myself, that's handy! I can carry this grumpy part in my pocket every day, keep her close, love her up—after all she's very adorable.

Then I landed back in my body but soon let out a shriek: I saw above me the rear end of a cockatoo and felt splatters on my face. I yelled to Alex, 'That cockie just shat in my face!'

'It's okay, it's just moving around and all the berries and debris are falling down. It's not shit, Mum.'

Crisis averted, I soon realised that I felt exhilarated. 'People with depression have to do this,' I told Alex. I felt completely reset. I felt like I could start my life anew.

I decided I'd stay the night at my mother's and dismissed Alex to his evening.

I lay alone, with my valley view, content. My body, as usual, felt hopelessly heavy and, for many hours, it would be impossible to stand up. Yet whereas on previous trips I'd felt frustrated and impatient with this post-trip feeling, this time was different. I was in nature and it had never looked so beautiful. I surrendered to the deep rest and felt a peace and serenity, as I watched how the summer breeze made the trees dance and the leaves flutter. I marvelled at the irony: I've been crisscrossing the planet only to discover the most beautiful place is in my childhood home.

Apart from meeting my grumpy old lady part, there had not been many 'takeaways' from the trip, yet I felt blissful, and I knew my body would feel lighter than ever once the heaviness subsided. Takeaways feed and appease the mind but sometimes it's the body's turn. I knew I'd released blockages, I just didn't know exactly what. I had a feeling, given the setting of my childhood home, that the releases related to my birth family and childhood experiences, as the cheeky face of my sister, a self-described 'committed Christian', had appeared to me many times throughout the trip, as if to say, 'Are you done yet with all these silly trips?'.

That evening

When darkness began to set in, I returned to the house and sought out my mother. She'd been aware I'd taken 'a medicine' in her backyard, but I'd spared her the inconvenient detail that it was LSD. I'd withheld from her most of the details of my ten trips to date, but I'd decided in the last few weeks that I needed to assure her that I was safe. I also wanted her to understand more about my project.

'I was thinking,' I asked Mum, 'maybe tonight you and I could watch a documentary together called *How To Change Your Mind* about psychedelics. It might give you some assurance that what I'm doing is safe.'

'Yes, I *have* wondered a bit about the safety,' she agreed.

Together we watched that first gripping episode about the history of LSD. To my surprise, Mum didn't grab the remote when the next episode, which was about psilocybin, rolled around.

'You don't have to watch it if you don't want to, Mum.'

'No, it's interesting.'

She asked me some questions and gave me a chance to share about my journey. The next day we watched the episodes about MDMA and then mescaline. I felt relieved that my mother could now understand what I'd been up to and wondered why I hadn't thought to watch the documentaries with her months ago.

Lying in a bed in my childhood home that night, my newly discovered part summoned my attention.

'Not so fast,' blurted the grumpy old lady.

'What's the problem?' I asked her.

'I find this whole idea of a cartoon character you keep in your pocket condescending. I don't want to be your cutesy pocket toy. It's offensive. I feel trivialised. I'm complex but you don't take me seriously.'

She was right. I'd always hated when young people saw older people as 'cute' and 'sweet'. It reduced them to soft toys, overlooked their achievements and potentially stole some of their hard-earned dignity. All the same, her appearance in my trip would start a working relationship with my irritable part. It was time to learn about her burdens so I could release them. I'd locate her in my body and use any sensations to help the investigation. Over the following days I engaged in the investigation and discovered—excuse the cliché—Daddy Issues. The inquiry took me back to raging arguments with my father as a teenager, when I'd felt dangerous extremes of irritation. Enough said.

Integration with Dr Max

I described the details of my second LSD trip to Dr Max, saving the best for last.

'I'm pretty sure you'll like this bit.' I smiled.

I told him about the gift to my Parts Therapy: discovering the grumpy old lady, about how she didn't want me to trivialise her as a cute pocket toy and about how this part may have been born when I was a teenager fighting with my father.

Dr Max was excited: 'Sarah, this is a major breakthrough. Your trip has created an opening to do some really important work. Do you feel like you're ready to explore that irritable part and see what more she has to say to you?'

I was ready, and so began the transition from talking about Internal Family Systems therapy to putting it into practice and engaging in conversations with parts. The aim of investigating a part is to learn to love it, gain its trust in the Self and allow it to unburden. The Self witnesses what the part wants to show it. Throughout the process, Dr Max became a 'parts-detector' and we identified four other parts that wanted to protect me from investigating the irritable part:

The Hedonist: this part wanted to avoid the whole project by seeking something more fun like a joke or a story.
The Dissociator: this part kept losing concentration and saying 'Sorry, I went blank, what was the question again?'
The Panicker: this part was scared of the irritable part and had always asked questions like, 'Why can't I control the irritation?', 'What if other people can perceive the irritation in me?', 'Why can't I be a nicer person?'.
The Sad Orphan: This was the exile who lived down in the dark dungeons, slumped over a table in her despondency. The irritable part existed to protect the Sad Orphan. After all, anger and irritation feel more empowering than sadness. The Sad Orphan constantly cried over all her failures to connect deeply with others. She was lonely and bereft.

Dr Max encouraged me to show respect for all these parts, to thank them for trying to protect me but also to ask each of them if they'd step aside for a short while so that the Self and Dr Max could focus on working with the irritable part. Dr Max then asked the irritable part all kinds of questions so that it could finally feel heard and understood after all those years of being repressed by the Panicker. He finished by asking me to tell the irritable part that the work had only just begun, that we were at the beginning of a process and not to expect permanent relief from the burdens just yet. I committed to some ways to work with this part in Dr Max's absence: spend some time with it during, and outside of, meditation, chat with it often, send it love or journal about it.

I came up with images for each of the parts I discovered so that I could call an image of a part to mind during daily life, if I needed to have a quick chat with one or offer reassurance from the Self. The long-term aim, after parts have unburdened, is to give them new roles. I've found parts more than ready to tell me about the new role they'd like to play. Some, that formed at a young age, just want to be playful, others want to offer understanding to parts in others who suffer similar struggles.

It may, at first glance, seem self-indulgent, or overly self-focused, to include all this information about the parts I've identified in myself. However, any spiritual or emotional journey teaches us that no one is special. Everyone has traces, to varying degrees, of the parts I found in myself. To identify and heal them in yourself helps you understand, and be patient with, such parts in others. After all, as LSD in particular taught me, everyone out there is a part of me. I am them. They are me. Separation is a delusion.

At the end of our session, Dr Max asked, 'So how are you finding Internal Family Systems therapy?'

'I'm finding it really useful,' I told him. 'Buddhism taught me the value of self-compassion at a general, or global, level but

Parts Therapy helps me to do a complete inventory, to uncover any hidden corners that I've failed to love. It's like going through my character with a fine-tooth comb to discover any orphans that need some love.'

With increased awareness and familiarity of my inner parts, the therapy paved the way for a lot more answers to Carlos's question, 'Who is experiencing this?'

'And if you do end up dating again,' Dr Max added, 'after some Parts Therapy, you'll hopefully have become the primary carer for your parts. I'm experienced as a couple's therapist and can tell you that so many relationships fail because people expect their partner to redeem them, to love all the exiled parts that they never managed to love by themselves. A partner, though, can only ever be a secondary carer otherwise we'll have unrealistic expectations of them.'

19

DMT near Newcastle

An opportunity for me to smoke DMT arose through a friend, Mike, who I'd met a few months back at an information day about psychedelic medicine. We'd stayed in close touch, bonding over time over our mutual fascination with psychedelics. He'd become a valuable mentor on my psychedelic journey and his knowledge had helped me more than once. This 35-year-old, soon father-to-be, woke at 5 a.m. every day to read books about psychedelics, for an hour or more, and he, too, had almost finished writing a book about them.

As with 5-MeO-DMT, the effects of regular DMT begin almost instantly and don't last long, 45 minutes at the most. Once it's over, there's no dizziness, disorientation or even fatigue—which is why some refer to it as 'the businessman's lunch'. No need to set a whole day aside as you do with all the other psychedelics, or nurse a hangover the next day.

I'd tried 5-MeO-DMT, otherwise known as Bufo, back in Portugal, but regular DMT, dimethyltryptamine, has different effects and is known for the frequency of encounters with otherworldly beings. I'd been fortunate to have an encounter with Kuan Yin, the Buddhist goddess of compassion, while on the Bufo retreat even though it was regular DMT that provided the best chance of meeting an entity.

As mentioned in chapter 12, DMT is a component of ayahuasca where the shamans combine DMT with the *Banisteriopsis caapi* vine to enable the DMT to last four hours instead of a few minutes. DMT abounds in plants such as acacia, or types of wattle trees in Australia, but also in animals, sea creatures and even the human brain. Both Bufo and regular DMT affect the serotonin receptors of the brain.

Mike

Mike's psychedelic journey began when he was seventeen years old, one afternoon, after he ran into an older cousin in the street of his small town in Eastern Europe. The cousin was in a rush but placed a bag of mushrooms in Mike's hands and suggested he try them. Mike didn't know anything about mushrooms and chomped them down, alternating with his chocolate bar to improve the taste. He now believes he took between 15 and 20 grams, many times a normal dose. Over the next fourteen hours, Mike experienced almost everything it's possible to experience on a psychedelic journey, starting with pulsating trees that were 'fully alive', feelings of connection to nature, visions of man's exploitation of nature, ecstatic love, entities, demons, ego dissolution, terror, deep peace, memories from childhood and vomiting. By nightfall he was profoundly lost in a dark forest, and terrified. It took him a while to overcome his terror and realise that the entity who had repeatedly appeared—with a human body and an owl's face—was using hand signals to point Mike in the direction of home.

After that trip, Mike had no desire to touch any psychedelics for another ten years. The story reminded me of that of mycologist Paul Stamets who, as an eighteen-year-old, took a massive dose of psilocybin and spent his trip in a forest, up a tree during a violent storm, from where he was permanently cured of a debilitating stutter.[1]

My attempted DMT trip

Mike offered to hold a DMT ceremony for me at a beautiful lookout in a national park near his home just outside the city of Newcastle. He'd advised me to eat no meat, or sugar, in the week beforehand, and to meditate as much as possible. Eventually, one Saturday night he treated me to a ceremony complete with the burning sage, shamanic music and ancient rituals with fire and smoke that had become familiar to me.

Mike loaded a pipe with what looked like tiny rocks resembling solidified earwax and presented the pipe to me three times: 10 micrograms, then 20, then 30. I sucked the smoke from the pipe, however, I felt a strong pain in my throat. I managed to take some of the smoke down into my lungs, but I coughed and spluttered. This activated my inner hypochondriac who felt certain I was doing irreversible damage to my throat tissues, but I persevered through each dose. On 10 micrograms, I felt a few minutes of relaxation and an inner stillness. On the 20 micrograms, my body felt the familiar cushiony, pillowy, plump feeling I'd experienced on past trips. I saw some colourful, swirling shapes and a male presence at my side, a human, ministering to me with what looked like chopsticks but it was only a vague, blurry impression. On the 30 micrograms, nothing at all happened, perhaps because I hadn't held it down long enough, or had coughed it all away. We tried the 30 micrograms again: my body experienced the delicious, anaesthetised feeling once more and I saw geometrical patterns, but that's all.

The problem seemed to be that I'd never been a smoker so had trouble taking the smoke down into my lungs and holding it for enough time. I hadn't had the same problem with 5-MeO-DMT in Portugal but 5-MeO is supposed to be four or six times stronger than regular DMT.[2] Nor had Dr Rick Strassman's DMT study participants, who we'll hear about later in this chapter, had this problem as they'd received DMT intravenously.

After my turn, Mike, who was highly experienced with DMT, took a mere 10 micrograms and during his ten-minute trip managed to dance, and laugh, with a joyful Buddha entity. He advised that next time I might need to line up a few pipes and take multiple inhalations in order to 'break through', the expression DMT users employ to describe entry into another dimension.

I'm not sure DMT will be my thing given it's so much easier for me to drink a psychedelic tea, but maybe I should keep an open mind. Mike said that DMT was a definite favourite due to its power and intensity. He reported that he'd consistently seen serpent entities on most of his DMT trips and had long wondered what the serpents wanted to convey to him. On one trip the serpents finally spoke to him:

A huge, brightly coloured serpent came into sight from the right and then another identical serpent from the left. They met in the centre of the room and merged to form a face, which focused on me. The face resembled a skull before morphing into an alien. I was speechless, so shocked by the show that I almost forgot to breathe. It was the most extraordinary entity I've ever encountered and I've seen a lot of entities during my trips. I felt fear.

The Face said: 'Fear and anger make you weak.'

'Who are you?' I asked.

'Birth and death,' replied the Face, 'being and nonbeing, light and darkness, self and other, love and fear.'

'What makes you think I'm fearful and angry?' I asked.

'The essence of your energy is unambiguous,' replied the Face.

The face separated into two serpents again, one slithered away to the right, the other to the left.

It's funny, Mike never struck me as the slightest bit fearful and angry. Maybe the serpents encounter had sorted him out well before I'd met him.

Entities in the hands of scientists

The research of psychiatrist Dr Rick Strassman who wrote the book *DMT: The Spirit Molecule*, suggested DMT can provide a powerful mystical experience. Likewise, an Australian study found 75.5 per cent of 121 respondents who'd taken DMT reported an increase in psychospiritual insight despite almost three-quarters claiming no religious affiliation.[3]

It's no secret that, on DMT, one is highly likely to meet with a goddess, a spirit animal or even an elf or a clown. One study from prestigious Johns Hopkins University surveyed 2,500 people who'd tried DMT and found that 50 per cent of them had encountered an otherworldly being. Furthermore, 80 per cent of those agreed that meeting an entity had 'altered their fundamental conception of reality' and 69 per cent of them claimed they'd received a message from the entity. Nineteen per cent said they'd received a prediction about the future from their entity. Intriguingly, 72 per cent stated that they continued to believe in the existence of their entity after their trip.[4] More than half of participants who'd identified as atheists before their DMT journey no longer did. The experience of Beatle Paul McCartney, back when the Beatles were still together, supports this data, according to a 2018 article, 'Drug session showed me "huge vision of God", reveals Paul McCartney'—the drug being DMT.[5]

Dr Rick Strassman was the first academic to gain US government approval and funding for new psychedelic research following Nixon's ban in 1970. Dr Strassman had been an experienced psychonaut while at university and was keen to discover how DMT might help people. From 1990 to 1995, after a two-decade drought in research,

Dr Strassman was able to inject over 50 research subjects with 400 doses of DMT.[6]

He could never have imagined, however, the results of his research—more than half of the subjects met a nonhuman life form—and the reader is left feeling sympathy for a man of science who felt way out of his depth in a world of mysticism, other realms and entities, variously described as 'beings', 'aliens', 'guides', 'helpers', 'clowns, reptiles, mantises, bees, spiders, cacti, and stick figures'. As Dr Strassman put it: 'I was neither intellectually nor emotionally prepared for the frequency with which contact with beings occurred in our studies, nor the often utterly bizarre nature of these experiences.'

Particularly baffling to the doctor was the number of subjects who recounted experiences resembling alien abduction.

> . . . The highly intelligent beings of this 'other' world are interested in the subject, seemingly ready for his or her arrival and wasting no time in 'getting to work' . . . Their business appeared to be testing, examining, probing, and even modifying the volunteer's mind and body . . . several subjects felt a benevolent attempt on the beings' part to improve us individually or as a race.

Such results led Dr Strassman to hypothesise that the DMT produced by our own brains, without the help of any drug, has caused people to believe they were abducted by aliens and for that experience to feel particularly real for them.

Dr Strassman noted, however, that all the subjects rejected any theories he presented to explain an entity encounter—a dream? some kind of brain mechanism?—as, for each of them, the experience was 'more real than real'. Podcaster Joe Rogan narrates a documentary on YouTube, *DMT: The Spirit Molecule*, released in 2010, where some of the research subjects recount, wide-eyed and excited, sometimes more than twenty years since their DMT sessions, their experience of another realm brimming with entities.

Dr Strassman was anything but excited at these discoveries:

> As the years passed, I began feeling a peculiar anxiety about listening to volunteers' accounts of their first high-dose DMT sessions. It was as if I didn't want to hear them. These psychotherapeutic, near-death, and mystical sessions repeatedly reminded me of their ineffectiveness in effecting any real change. I wanted to say, 'That's very interesting, but now what? To what purpose?' By extension, these sessions' lack of lasting impact began eroding the basic foundations of my motivation for performing this type of research. Additionally, the reports of contact with invisible worlds and their inhabitants, while utterly amazing, left me grasping at conceptual straws as to their reality and meaning.

As the first study for twenty years, he was obliged to keep risks low so could only use 'normal' volunteers rather than real patients, and his volunteers had to be experienced with psychedelics. Eventually, he decided that therapy should accompany the psychedelic, but he lacked the resources to provide it. In an email exchange I had with him he explained: 'The success of our study—gaining funding, approval, and safely generating and publishing valuable data—caught the research world unprepared. Thus, it was difficult to build out our research team with additional chemists and pharmacologists, and cognitive, psychotherapy, and brain imaging clinical scientists.'

More recent researchers of the effects of DMT have found even greater frequency of encounters with otherworldly beings, 33 of 36 participants in one study, albeit with participants who were experienced DMT users. Unlike Dr Strassman, the researchers identified lasting impacts of entity encounters. One was the wellbeing that comes from increased 'psychological flexibility' given that the encounters 'call into question one's axioms of reality'.[7] This was certainly a lasting impact of psychedelics that I'd experienced myself: once we start questioning our basic assumptions about reality, old rigidities in other areas of our thinking can fall away.

20

Mescaline and ketamine in Sydney

The mescaline trips of both writers Michael Pollan and Aldous Huxley were eyes-open experiences, for Pollan, marvelling at the natural world or, in the case of Huxley, at the folds of his trousers, the spines of his book collection and the legs of a chair.[1] They portray a medicine that allows them to engage in a deeper relationship with the present moment, to perceive more of their surroundings than they routinely notice, and to recognise the miracle of the everyday.

Anthropologists write of artefacts proving that Native Americans have taken mescaline in ceremonies for 6000 years.[2] Consumed as a tea, or in a powdered form, it is the product of two alternative cacti: peyote or San Pedro (in South America, where the sacred cactus grows in the Andes region, the name is *wachuma*). Peyote takes a decade to grow and is scarce, so it's deemed best to leave it for the indigenous peoples who have a historical relationship with it. San Pedro, on the other hand, grows quickly and poses no sustainability issues.

Mescaline and I didn't get off to a good start. I'd attended a picnic in Sydney for people interested in plant medicines where a young man had handed out pieces of San Pedro cactus. I tried to make a tea and within one minute, I'd stabbed myself in the thumb with a cactus spine and part of it lodged under my skin where a blister would fester for weeks. I boiled the cactus tea for many hours but every recipe I found online seemed inconsistent and confusing—some made it seem simple, others something only a chemist could cook. When I eventually drank my tea, I felt nothing more than mildly drunk. Fail.

I decided to buy some. I had joined the mailing list of a man outside Sydney who ran ayahuasca retreats and sold a few plant medicines. People spoke highly of him. I soon received a bottle of pre-made cactus juice in the mail. The bottle said a strong dose was 80 to 100 milligrams. My plan was to take 80 milligrams and boost it by 20 at the three-hour point.

I'd decided to use my mother's backyard again for my mescaline trip as I loved the view with all the tall trees in the valley. Now that I'd experienced more than ten trips, I felt that having my mother rattling around in the house nearby was all the trip-sitting I needed. Mescaline takes two or three hours to act. The nausea after half an hour was vile and lasted over an hour but it did eventually pass. At least I didn't vomit.

Mescaline trip

As with my LSD trips, the trip lasted only around six hours instead of the twelve people often speak of, leaving me with the usual post-trip lethargy for many hours. As with LSD, I experienced nothing like the love and euphoria I had experienced with MDMA, psilocybin and ayahuasca but still enjoyed a fascinating, fun experience.

Perhaps due to the short amount of time since the last trip along with the common setting of my childhood home, both medicines, LSD and mescaline, gave me similar messages and impressions and defied a narrative structure. For mescaline, in particular, there could be no trip report.

As with LSD, once the medicine took effect, I could easily become confused about who I was, such as when I found myself asking: *Am I my sister right now? I seem to be in her head. Have I actually been her all along?* This is not an uncommon experience when taking LSD and I'd had this 'I am you, you are me' message several times now. It seemed to be a recurring theme in my recent trips. The words seem so lifeless on the page, yet during a trip such messages feel easy to understand, obvious even, and important.

My sense of identity, all sense of being that woman called Sarah with all her history and her roles in life, went on extended leave again. During the peak of the trip when I shuddered violently, I had the strong impression that 'Sarah' was absent so that my body could be used as a processing centre for the traumas of people through the ages. As with LSD, I had many visions from history—I trudged alongside refugee women wearing old-world clothing as we hurried along stormy, windswept beaches. At points, I had a sense, as happened on psilocybin, that my shuddering body was being used to process the traumas of the raped women throughout history. It's tempting to wonder if I'd revisited scenes from a past life. Stan Grof would certainly endorse such an interpretation or, alternatively, that I'd been immersed in the 'collective unconscious' of humanity.

Through a stream of visions, I received messages that sound preachy but, during the trip, had felt important: you are not inferior, nor superior, to anyone—such feelings are illusory; you've probably been wrong, ego-inflated, and insensitive all those times you argued the rightness of your views with others; stop privileging discursive thought and reasoning—prioritise the free flow of love between all humans.

As always, I enjoyed the trip, which had felt like an illuminating adventure, but I was frustrated at how much I'd forgotten by the time it was over. I'd wonder if being the type of person who almost never remembers their dreams on waking might correlate with forgetfulness following a trip. I detected a pattern in many of my trips: once the journey took off I'd say to myself, *Oh yes, I remember this feeling, how could I ever have forgotten?* Later in the trip I'd realise: *there's no way I'm going to remember much of this.* They all seemed to defy the narrative structure we crave for meaning-making. I remembered Carlos and Fanny saying that your Soul remembers, even if the small egoic mind forgets.

The eyes-open experiences of Pollan and Huxley on mescaline, marvelling at whatever they gazed upon, were no guide to my experience. Yet again, the force of the medicine saw me lying down, eyes firmly shut.

On the three trips I'd taken as a single woman, I'd experienced, on the comedown, a yearning for a loving partner to trip with. I'd wondered before the trips if the medicine would give me a message like, 'You're strong enough to live alone—stop all this craving a partner', 'Dedicate a year to being alone, to finding yourself', 'You don't need a man to complete you', but somehow I emerged from my trips more determined to find someone.

After mescaline

The day after my mescaline trip, I felt hungover, and out of sorts, and even deeply depressed for a few hours—so much for an after-glow. It was my mindset. I'd resumed internet dating, which is notoriously hard on anyone's mental health. The expansive, spacious mind that psychedelics fashion, shrinks to the size of a sultana as you swipe your way through endless unsuitable profiles. Necessarily, you become judgemental of your fellow humans again, old biases resurrected, as the poor man in each dating profile is too this, or too that. When you finally find a profile that inspires hope, the recipient doesn't respond to your witty message, as is their absolute right, of course, but it activates all my old rejection sensitivity.

My exiles—particularly the one who feels uncared for, and especially the one that feels 'not good enough'—arc up: *I told you I was ugly but you didn't listen! I'll never find the one, Why didn't he respond—I know he looked at my profile—what didn't he like? This has happened five times now!!* And on and on: *Maybe all that positive feedback Luke gave me about my physical appearance was incorrect? Maybe eyelash-extensions will make someone love me.* Worst of all, you feel a sense that you've betrayed yourself. In an act of self-commodification, you reduce all your nuance and complexity to a dating profile and post it on the Net for sale to the highest bidder.

It would be fair to ask what I was doing on a dating app, when I was supposed to be diligently 'integrating' my mescaline experience through attentive self-care. The thing is: the misery-machines we call dating apps are addictive. Like playing the pokies, it's hard to stop checking your phone and searching, in case the big win is but one swipe away.

So, the day after mescaline, I sat my depressed self on my meditation cushion to calm down and process the rejections. I listened to those exiles—*nobody likes me, I'm ugly, I'm a loser baby, so why don't you kill me, et cetera*—and comforted them. How easy it is to cede control to the exiles, but I told them the Self was back now, would listen to them, comfort them but take over the driver's seat.

It worked.

I was amazed that by the time I stood up from the cushion my mood had soared into something positive. I was getting good at comforting my exiles. I would clearly need to put some boundaries up around app use: while on the apps, I'd need to monitor my exiles with unstinting self-awareness and also allocate stretches of time for digital detoxing.

Given the neuroplasticity of our brains, after a psychedelic journey one is prone to be 'suggestible' for a few days. This is positive, of course, if we use our suggestibility for good and not evil. I've even heard the advice to avoid researching conspiracy theories after taking psychedelics, an activity that could consume a lot of your time and alienate you from your friends. I remembered this advice a couple of days after taking mescaline, when I found myself feverishly investigating everything I could find about reincarnation. After all, during my trips I'd found myself in scenes from centuries ago, playing historic characters. My memories were only vague and dreamlike but a few of the scenes had stayed with me.

I knew my former self would shake her head in disapproval at my recent interest in reincarnation. I knew certain friends would decide I'd become kooky. For a few moments I wondered to myself if I had, indeed, become kooky. Yet I found so much of the evidence for reincarnation undeniable. Why were there thousands of thoroughly researched accounts of children who had in-depth and detailed knowledge about a deceased person, about the specific details of another life? Sometimes a child even mysteriously knew a foreign language or had recurring nightmares about a violent death, which they constantly revisited in their play. Scientifically minded researchers had collected plenty of stories and produced several books. It's true that nobody understands the 'mechanisms' by which reincarnation could happen but there's a lot we humans don't know. I started loading my e-reader with the books providing evidence: autobiographies, anthologies and story collections—all written by seemingly sensible people.

Admittedly, I wanted reincarnation to be true for all the meaning and enchantment it could add to my life, and just because I want something to be true doesn't necessarily rule it out of possibility. If reincarnation was true, then all the suffering of our current lives could be useful to teach us lessons and prepare us for all our future lives.

A brief, but memorable, moment had occurred on the psilocybin retreat that felt informed by reincarnation. One of the women on the retreat was physically beautiful, bubbly, confident, successful and brilliant. Everyone, especially the men, loved her. I did too, she was irresistible, but a part of me also felt sad: how come *she* gets such an easy ride through life? How I'd love to have that kind of self-confidence, constantly affirmed by everyone around me. When the peak of my psilocybin trip had finished and my eyes were open, I looked over at her, sitting across the room from me. An inner voice said: 'Just let her have a turn'. In that moment, it was as if I knew, on some deep level, that in past incarnations she'd struggled, and that in future incarnations, she would struggle again.

Ketamine

Ketamine is not, technically, a psychedelic but a member of the class of drugs called 'dissociatives'—it leads to a detachment from reality. On a high dose the effects are similar to those of psychedelics so people speak of it as one. Unlike the psychedelics, however, ketamine can be addictive and long-term overuse—which I wasn't planning on—can cause all kinds of physical problems such as 'ketamine bladder syndrome'. I don't want to know what that is.

Developed in the 1960s as an anaesthetic, intravenous ketamine is legal in medical settings, in the United States and various European countries, to treat a range of mental health problems, particularly depression, but also addictions and eating disorders. Today hundreds of ketamine clinics dot the map of the United States. In Australia, ketamine treatment is expensive and only available from registered clinics for hard-to-treat depression. Professor David Nutt celebrated ketamine in his guidebook published in 2023 *Psychedelics*, as 'the first pharmacologically novel antidepressant in over 30 years'.[3]

It would not be unfair to say, however, that ketamine has less therapeutic potential than psilocybin. Maybe it's only logical given a ketamine trip lasts around an hour compared to psilocybin's average of six hours. I attended a webinar organised by Mind Medicine Australia (more about MMA in chapter 21) with psychiatrist and researcher, Reid Robison, who has guided thousands of ketamine therapy journeys (and I was interested to note, uses Internal Family Systems therapy). He said, comparing ketamine to psilocybin:

> You don't have as much built-in insight as you do with a high dose of psilocybin. Ketamine can still be a profound mystical experience. It can be a state of consciousness where someone downloads some of the most meaningful insights of their life but, on average, across big numbers of people, I would say you have to work a little harder as a therapist to help people make sense of it . . . People, fairly commonly, will say, 'that was strange', or 'weird', or they don't even know how to describe it.[4]

He then produced a fascinating graph, from the research of neuroscientist Gül Dölen (known for her MDMA study of octopuses mentioned in chapter 10), which showed that the window of neuroplasticity, for 'malleability and learning', was two days for ketamine, two weeks for psilocybin and MDMA, and three weeks for LSD.[5]

The effects of ketamine take only minutes to arise and the mood-lifting afterglow can last several days. While at low doses the effects can feel similar to alcohol, such as deep relaxation, high doses provide the opportunity to enter the 'K-hole'—which terrifies some and delights others. In the K-hole, you can lose your sense of self, dissolve into your surroundings and leave reality far behind.[6] I would soon learn, the hard way, that while many adore the effects of ketamine, some will be persecuted by them.

When the ketamine arrived in the post, I used a drug test, where I dropped a ketamine crystal into some yellow liquid, which momentarily flashed red to indicate the presence of ketamine. This is worth doing given the new drug-testing facility in Canberra found only six out of fourteen samples of ketamine submitted to them were actually ketamine.[7] The day prior to taking it, I 'sniffed' (I can't bring myself to say 'snorted') a few pinches, or what users call 'bumps', to test my reaction. The low dose made me feel pleasantly drunk: I couldn't walk in a straight line, but rather than the heavy feeling alcohol produces, I felt light and floaty.

Ketamine at Trish's house

The next day I cycled to Trish's house at around 11 a.m. I felt less precious about guarding my mindset from chatter, for what was supposed to be a one-hour trip, so I chatted with Trish and told her what I knew about ketamine and what to expect. I'd go first so that Trish could trip-sit me, and vice versa. I used my mortar and pestle to crush the fine crystals into a powder before I stood in front of a mirror (for guidance), dipped a butter knife into the mix, and sniffed a series of 'bumps'. I'm told young recreational users crush the crystals between two credit cards before sniffing it through a bank note, or sniffing it off a house key, which all sounded unhygienic to my middle-aged ears. The sniffing was painless as I could control the amount each time. The effects came on within a minute.

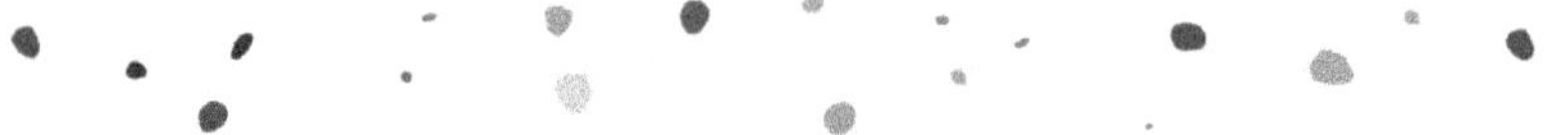

Still standing up, I close my eyes and there's a black-and-white cartoon of a pair of dancers on a checkerboard floor. I haven't even sat down yet but bend over into yoga's ragdoll pose. It feels like a perfectly comfortable position to trip in for a minute or two but then I make my way to the floor, which feels like a challenging movement—how exactly do I reach the floor from here?

I'm pleased that this trip feels strong. I feel several versions of happiness in succession, but the one that settles for the longest is a cool, calm happiness, not euphoria with its high energy, but a certainty that everything in this moment is just right. For a while there are no visuals, only twinkling white light and this quiet happiness. I feel the floor kindly supporting my back, and the couch snugly supporting my upraised calves. Why did I ever worry about a thing in my life? Everything's wonderful.

The visuals return, featuring painted images from the colours found in sunsets, that pass me as if on invisible conveyer belts. As they pass, I hear 'the small mind' producing its habitual comments and acknowledge that this is just what the mind will always do no matter what's happening—when are we moving onto the next thing? Why can't I be pretty? Why can't I find a partner? How can I get rid of bad moods and make my life perfect? I understand that I don't have to identify with any of it. The mantra I hear a hundred times, 'It doesn't matter, it doesn't matter, none of it matters'.

Now I'm a man with a beard. It feels nice to have a beard and I stroke my face watching myself, or man-me, from above. Still from above, I see myself turn into a painting of Sarah who repeatedly hugs herself and rubs her arms. 'Love this girl!' comes the message, 'she's very precious'. I see a stream of photos of myself, including one of me ziplining through a tree canopy. I look deeply happy in all the photos and I feel accepting of my image, happy for her happiness, instead of critical of the photo.

When it's over, within an hour, I feel tired, and spaced out, but none of the heaviness I felt after LSD. I have no idea if I was in the so-called K-hole, but if I was, I liked it. I reflected that it was such a treat to visit the unfamiliar worlds I'd visited in my early trips with all the pretty colours, patterns and unexpected images. With LSD and mescaline, I'd travelled back hundreds of years but, with a couple of fleeting exceptions, such as the pelican princess, most of the visuals had been earth-based.

I announce to Trish, 'All done! It was magical. I loved it. You are in for a real treat, girl. I'm excited for you! Let's get you sorted'.

After sniffing a few bumps Trish announced, 'It's coming on', and took herself to her bedroom where I'd intermittently check on her. I sat on a couch feeling vague and spacey but as though I could resume normal activities within the hour.

When Trish emerged from her bedroom after an hour she said, 'I don't feel so well', and walked to the toilet where I heard her vomit. It was, apparently, her second purge.

'I don't think this one's for me,' she said, grimacing. 'I felt like I had a chemical inside me.'

I don't know if Trish was still affected by some alcohol she'd drunk two nights previously with some visiting houseguests, but I gave her a spiel.

'There's a school of thought,' I launched, 'that vomiting when you take psychedelics is purging impurities that are holding you back in life. I know a retreat facilitator up north who calls vomiting *getting well*.'

She probably wanted to slap me but managed to restrain herself.

I soon cycled home at around 3 p.m. and texted Trish throughout the evening but she remained nauseous. I felt guilty. I'd assumed, after our LSD experience, that she'd need a dose larger than mine. Sniffing ketamine provides the option of taking it gradually and boosting over time but I'd been so excited after my experience that I encouraged her to waste no time and load up with a similar dose to mine. I searched the internet throughout the afternoon and found that some sites mentioned vomiting as the sign of a ketamine overdose.

Yes.

I became haunted by images of Trish attending emergency and of me having to explain to her loved ones what had happened.

At 9 p.m. I texted again:

Any improvement?

Trish replied:

Yes, bit better now thanks—got a feeling I should've done the gradual approach (laughing and crying emoji) went into it fast and the full-body reaction was a surprise despite you prepping me (gritted teeth emoji). At one point I wasn't sure if my mind would make it back, it was soooo bizarre, I kept trying to enjoy it but it was like I was lost inside my mind.

Me:

Sounds like you k-holed.

Trish:

I felt like I was experiencing infinity and travelling on and on and I wondered how my body knew to breathe. It was interesting for the first half but then the nausea hit.

On my immediate post-trip high it had been beyond me to imagine that Trish would not experience the bliss I had. Lesson learned.

Despite enjoying my trip, I can't say I experienced much of an afterglow in the following days. The next day, I woke at 4 a.m. and felt extremely tired all day, which is never good for my mood. I also blame the slings and arrows of internet dating, which continued to punish me, with rejections flowing in both directions. I kept repeating the mantra from my trip, 'it doesn't matter', which helped me keep a sense of proportion, but I knew it was also important to allow space for my exiles to sulk rather than suppress them.

I may have been more successful at exploiting the 48-hour window of neuroplasticity that ketamine provides if I'd been seeing an integration therapist, but my appointments with the popular Dr Max were too many weeks apart. It reminded me that for psychedelics to heal or transform, the therapy was important, whether with a professional, a support group or a wise friend. Of course, many of us have the inner resources to do our own therapy, so I kept reading books, particularly about Internal Family Systems therapy, so that I could be my own therapist and maximise the benefit of the trip.

Integration, integration, integration.

21

Psychedelic-assisted psychotherapy

In our post-COVID world, where demand for mental health treatment is at an all-time high, psychedelics are likely to be the future. Back in the fifties and sixties, with a thousand research papers to support them, psychedelics were set to be the 'next big thing' in psychiatry.[1] Since Nixon's ban on psychedelic research back in 1970, millions have suffered, or even died by suicide, for want of adequate medication. The legal mental health medications that we've relied on, as we wait for the legalisation of psychedelics, can have a range of challenging side effects: they numb us emotionally, kill our libidos or trigger weight gain, to name a few.

The war on drugs saw a three-decade ban on all research, but research has well and truly resumed. The database of one advocacy group in the United States, Blossom Analysis,[2] indicates there are 305 trials of psychedelics under way around the world, conducted in some of the world's most prestigious universities. Thirty-eight trials are in Australia and New Zealand.[3]

It's common knowledge, in the world of psychedelics, that plenty of people, particularly veterans with post-traumatic stress disorder, have been prepared to seek help underground rather than spend years waiting for the laws to catch up with the research. While there are plenty of caring professionals and brave souls working underground, it's also an unregulated Wild West where the greedy, the ego-inflated or the predatory can lurk.

The night before I left for Amsterdam to attend my psilocybin retreat, a distinguished speaker visited the town hall two blocks from my home. Professor David Nutt, the neuropsychopharmacologist and pioneer in psychedelic research, who I have quoted many times throughout this book, would speak alongside a panel of experts and people affected by the Australian government's inertia about the need for access to psychedelic-assisted psychotherapy. I tend to protect myself with low expectations in the general course of life, so pictured twenty people attending, 50 at the most, but there were hundreds. The huge hall was full.

Professor Nutt would also gain an audience with the Therapeutic Goods Administration as they wrestled with their decision about whether to legalise psilocybin and MDMA for treatment-resistant depression and PTSD. The rest is history: from July 2023, Australia became the first country in the world to make the substances legal for medical purposes.

Meeting the co-founder of Mind Medicine Australia (MMA)

The non-profit organisation and charity Mind Medicine Australia advocates for psychedelic-assisted psychotherapy, and is the force behind Australia becoming the first country in the world to reclassify psilocybin and MDMA to allow suffering people access. Tania de Jong AM and Peter Hunt AM founded the organisation in 2019 and, yes, they are a married couple.

If Tania could be captured in one word, the word might be 'influential'. She's featured in lists such as the global Top 100 Most Influential People in Psychedelics, the Top 100 Most Influential Women in Australia and the 100 Most Influential Australian Entrepreneurs, also winning an Ernst & Young Entrepreneur of the Year award. She's a member of the Order of Australia for service to the arts and, has set up six businesses and four charities including Mind Medicine Australia. Oh, and she's a soprano who's performed in 40 countries, released seven albums with her singing group and six solo albums. She's a global speaker, including a TED Talk, and she's a prolific contributor of articles to our newspapers. This list is by no means complete. I don't know what the fuck I've being doing with *my* life. When I emailed Tania to request an interview, it felt like a miracle that she could spare me some time.

Tania would be in Sydney to sing and I treated myself to a second-row seat to watch the musical she'd produced, *Driftwood*, based on the memoir written by her mother. Tania played the part of her Holocaust-surviving grandmother, who happens to be the inventor of the foldable umbrella.

I met Tania in the lobby after the show. And waited for the streams of people to finish shaking her hand and chatting to her, then introduced myself and congratulated her on a moving performance.

'I could never have played the role of my grandmother,' Tania said, 'night after night like this, if I hadn't taken the medicines—I wouldn't have had the courage.'

As Tania's husband Peter describes her, she's a 'brilliant connector' and despite having just starred in a show, she took a moment to inquire about me.

'So what made you decide to write this particular book?'

'Apart from the selfish reasons,' I began, 'of pursuing my own curiosity and desire for adventure, I'm hyperaware of human suffering and I just think it's wrong that governments, through the war on drugs and prohibition, have separated us from a natural source of relief, and so many opportunities for personal growth. Humans, with or without a diagnosis, need to be reunited with what I see as their birthright, a psychedelic experience.'

'You're definitely right about the human suffering out there,' Tania replied. 'I receive heartbreaking emails from people in their fifties and sixties saying they'd love a few years with more light and meaning, without mental illness.'

'Not to mention,' I replied, 'all the people who have died by suicide, all over the world, for want of effective medication.'

We arranged to speak again over Zoom, a week later, when Tania had regained her energy after her performance season.

Interview with Tania de Jong

'The greatest achievement of Mind Medicine Australia,' I began, 'would have to be, of course, persuading the Australian Government to become the first country in the world to allow psilocybin for treatment-resistant depression and MDMA for PTSD. How on earth did you do that?'

'Yes, it's all very exciting. Mind Medicine Australia was instrumental in encouraging over 13,000 Australians, via our webinars and our mailing list, to write submissions to the Therapeutic Goods Administration.'

'Yes, I sent one!' I bleated.

'We also arranged for leading neuropsychopharmacologist Professor David Nutt to come out from Imperial College London and speak to 130 people at the TGA, and to other audiences in Australia, from the general public to clinicians, researchers and politicians.'

'Yes, I went to his public talk, which was certainly well-attended, and where I heard you sing for the opening of the event.'

'David is such an authority figure in the field with all the scientific data at his fingertips, so we're sure that really helped push the TGA over the line.'

'I've heard,' I said, 'that when you first tried psilocybin you were someone who never drank alcohol, or even tea and coffee, let alone psychedelic drugs. You were staunchly anti-drug.'

'Yes, I had no idea what it was like to be drunk, or in an altered state of consciousness, unless you count the high from singing, which I'd always described as my drug of choice,' Tania laughed.

'So how did you become involved in the world of psychedelics?'

'It all started after I read an article by Michael Pollan in the *New Yorker*, which I'd heard about through a blog by Tim Ferriss. The article was about research on end-of-life anxiety and the results were staggering.'

'Michael Pollan.' I nodded. 'He was my entrée as well.'

'So the end-of-life study found that after only two doses of psilocybin, 80 per cent of the cancer sufferers were largely cured of anxiety and depression and, importantly, they'd remained that way when followed up over four years later.[4] Anyway, one of the people in the study was the child of Holocaust survivors who, like me, had always felt the effects of that intergenerational trauma. My husband Peter had his own trauma as his father died by suicide when Peter was thirteen years old. So Peter and I travelled to the Netherlands where we met a guide and tried mushroom truffles—which are legal in that country. I was, of course, petrified in the lead-up at the idea of losing control.'

'So how did that go?'

'Impossible to describe but utterly life-changing—the sense of connection to the Self, to others, to the planet, the sense of oneness, the gratitude for life and for nature, even the increased acceptance for how things are—it took us a full year to integrate it all. We returned to the Netherlands a year later for another experience with the same guide and had an even more powerful multi-dimensional experience. I've felt so much healing, more love radiating from me, greater wholeness and wellness, and importantly, it set us on a course of self-development, as we worked through the insights we'd experienced. I feel as though it's increased my creativity, my energy. I have more moments of flow, or deep engagement, in all my work.'

'Wow. So how did Mind Medicine Australia come about?'

'We connected with some of the leaders in the field who told us that Australia was very behind, so we saw there was a gap to fill, and we understood firsthand the potential of these medicines. If psychedelics can provide an experience of connection, then they could be a powerful tool to help people with mental illness, which is so often caused by a sense of hopelessness, isolation and disconnection. Peter and I know, having set up a series of charities, that at the heart of most disadvantage lies mental illness. If we can help with that, it could help our other charities, and the whole charity sector, to help many more people feel a sense of belonging and lead healthier, happier and more meaningful lives.'

'And you knew that the current medicines have been pretty ineffective.'

'Yes! The existing treatments have a 30 to 35 per cent success rate for depression, and only 5 per cent for PTSD. Compare that to the findings from over 300 trials of a 60 to 80 per cent success rate after taking the medicines only two or three times along with psychotherapy. Depression treatment methods haven't substantially changed for decades and even if you recover, there's as much as an 80 per cent chance your illness will return. Don't forget the side effects and withdrawal symptoms as well. We aren't arguing that psychedelics will work for every single patient. However, people need options and it's a basic human right to have access to safe and effective medicine.'

'I know from attending your webinars that you see Australia as an urgent case for improvement in mental health.'

'Definitely. Australia has the second highest rates of mental illness in the world of OECD countries, second only to Icelanders who live in the cold and the dark for much of the year. Before the pandemic, one in five Australians experienced some type of mental illness. As for anti-depressants, one in seven adults, and one in four older people, were estimated to take them. Children as young as four are prescribed psychiatric medicines. How much more will the pandemic have increased these numbers? Some experts have warned us to expect an increase of 25 per cent in those numbers.'

'I've had a good look around the Mind Medicine Australia website, and you could spend a month there with all those podcasts, articles and resources, but I was particularly impressed by the sheer number of achievements. You're doing much more than just raising awareness. I read that Mind Medicine Australia have done a deal with a Canadian supplier and will supply the medicines to psychiatrists. On top of that, you've set up a fund so that people can donate to helping with the cost of the therapy for those who can't afford it.'

'Yes, the Patient Support Fund. A course of treatment could cost around $15,000—we don't know yet as it's still early days—but it's the cost of the therapy, rather than the medicine, that really adds up. Then again, we need to weigh this cost up against the cost of conventional medication and therapy for potentially the rest of a patient's life with current treatments, which do not lead to healing for the majority.'

The achievements of MMA are so numerous that I told Tania I'd check the website for the full list. After all of her work for

MMA and following her 45 Melbourne and Sydney performances of *Driftwood* she deserved a rest.

Given that nobody can access the newly legal medicines without therapy, Mind Medicine Australia has, to date, trained 360 mental health practitioners—psychiatrists, psychologists, psychotherapists, GPs and more, including Dr Max—in a world-class course they developed called the Certificate in Psychedelic-Assisted Therapies (CPAT). Hundreds more will do the training as future demand increases for the therapy, and clinical supervision of graduates is also set to occur.

In addition, MMA supports four different research trials including provision of free medicines. Their advocacy has secured 15 million dollars from the Australian Government to support psychedelic medicine research, the largest government grant for this purpose anywhere in the world. They have established 33 local chapters, all over the country, that run educational events and social get-togethers. The Holotropic Breathwork workshop I attended, for example, in chapter 9, was organised by their Sydney chapter.

I hoped that among Tania's many skills is delegation.

Healing stories

In 2021, Mind Medicine Australia published a book *Mind Medicine: Psychedelic healing stories from Australia*. To attract submissions from the psychedelic medicine community, they set up a webpage inviting anyone to send their healing story. Over a six-month period, the stories streamed in and they chose 54 for publication. The book is highly compelling, even though almost every story has the same plot points. Each person suffered from debilitating mental health problems—sixteen of the stories mention suicide—and almost everyone had 'tried everything', many providing a long list of different therapies that hadn't worked for them. Finally, they tried psychedelic medicine and experienced a healing beyond anything they'd ever hoped for. Most of them also emphasised the need to keep working on themselves after taking the medicine and acknowledged that the medicine wouldn't work without some commitment to integrate what they'd learned.

Here are a couple of abridged samples:

Simone Dowding, 49-year-old CEO—ayahuasca

Here I was, a successful entrepreneur living a millionaire lifestyle. I had made it! But something was missing. The success I had valued and strived my whole life for had left me empty and in a marriage that died in the process. I don't think anyone can describe the loss of a marriage . . . In the midst of all the trauma, change and never-ending tears something else dawns on you too.

I am now . . . alone.

In my aloneness, I grew afraid. The world had lost all meaning and I felt completely disconnected from everyone and everything. Nothing brought me joy and I was trapped in extreme suicidal ideations that left me unable to work and be social. My family was unable to understand me, and I was gradually losing all my friendships. Leaving me more disconnected and isolated.

. . . I went to every type of Western doctor and tried various medications.

Simone provides a long list of different therapies she tried including acupuncture, hypnosis, counselling and meditation. Eventually someone suggested ayahuasca and within three months she sat with a shaman deep in the Amazon jungle of Peru and drank the tea.

The first night was one of the most frightening nights of my life. I was confronted with all my grief and trauma and challenged to find my power within it. I felt the shaman and medicine, training me to be strong, resilient and face all my fears. By the end of that night, I had a sacred and profound initiation. I felt new, clean, and strong. Most importantly, I had been given the ability to dream again. But the greatest gift of all was that . . . I wanted to live.

I realised the key to my mental and spiritual health was to completely let go of my old life, my past, ancestral history, culture, trauma and subconscious programming. It was more than a psychological healing, though. I had awakened into something new. I profoundly connected with something greater than myself. The realisation had dawned on me that I was never alone. I have a peaceful acceptance of my past now, as painful as it was, and I realise that nothing happened by accident.

On my return from the Amazon I worked for World Vision Australia as the Head of Social Enterprise, which enabled me to economically empower women globally. I was then voted in the top 50 Business People of the Year in Australia by *Inside Business* magazine for my contribution to humanity. I am currently CEO of a national organisation and a guest lecturer for Monash University. Most importantly, I am a loving and present mum to my two gorgeous boys.

Big love, Sim.

Graeme Sudholz, 64-year-old relationship counsellor—MDMA and psilocybin

My trauma started from the moment I was born. As a young child, I lived in pure terror of my mother. On numerous occasions, she tried to stop me from crying by drowning me in the bath. She tried to suffocate me with a pillow on her last attempt and she was so close to being successful that time.

The terror from these experiences was held in my body and controlled every aspect of my life, regardless of how much energy and time I invested in trying to overcome my troubles. Sometimes, I would sit for days, frozen solid in terror. I could feel the terror and trauma, but only had brief and fleeting glimpses of what happened. This wreaked havoc on my intimate relationships and my first marriage, a 26-year relationship, ended in divorce.

After a suicide attempt, my counsellor 'threw' me into a workshop on emotional intelligence. At that workshop, I met Annette, my life partner and since then we have shared a passion for personal development, training and healing. Our unconscious and personal wounds drew us together and we became relationship counsellors, establishing a relationship counselling and tantra business together in 2005.

It took us twenty years in this space, to discover psychedelic-assisted therapy, and since our first experiences, we've had outstanding success in healing both as individuals and together as a couple.

I have experienced psychedelic-assisted therapy with MDMA, psilocybin, and a combination of both. Each has merit, and each has worked in different ways. Psilocybin helped me to unlock all those self-defeating beliefs that I relied on so heavily to avoid feeling my terrorised, traumatised self, and to instil healthy self-beliefs. My experience with MDMA allowed me to access the trauma held deep in my body, explore it without retraumatising myself, and let it go. I have been able to walk away from my trauma and leave it behind, permanently. Now I am free.

My intention in sharing this story is to bring attention to the deep healing available to us through psychedelic medicines. Everyone deserves the chance to experience psychedelic medicines, and to heal.

It's easy when reading all the healing stories to assume that psychedelics are wonder drugs that heal anyone and harm nobody. Yet as with any medicine, there will be those that aren't healed, and, in rare circumstances, those that are harmed. Mind Medicine Australia would argue, however, that anyone suffering from depression, or PTSD, should at least have the option to access the medicines with the best results according to the research to date.[5]

22

The future of psychedelics

As more of us see clearly the misinformation of the global war on drugs, curiosity about psychedelics grows. The renaissance is well under way and governments around the world increasingly legalise psychedelics as a mental-health treatment. Progressive countries, such as Portugal, some European countries and the odd state in the US, decriminalise them with many scientists backing these developments. The genie is out of the bottle, but it's important to reflect deeply on the form we want any new freedom to take.

On the psilocybin retreat, I met Alexander Beiner, who co-facilitates many retreats with Natasja. Soon after that retreat, he released a book *The Bigger Picture: How psychedelics can help us make sense of the world* in which he urges us not to limit psychedelics to any particular model. He worries that we'll lose the enormous potential for psychedelics to solve our global problems if we define them as only for mental health or only for spiritual searching.

> The risk is that big pharma, the well-being industry, and biomedical psychiatry create a narrative around what psychedelics are, who they are for, and how they are allowed to be used—which narrows their tremendous potential for social change.[1]

Dr Christopher Bache, who took LSD 73 times (back in chapter 16), would probably agree with Alexander's concerns about limiting the potential of psychedelics: he sought not personal healing, although that happened too, but an understanding of the universe.[2]

Beiner argues we need both 'churches and clinics' whether this means new churches for psychedelics or introducing them into existing churches in the hope of reinvigorating them. He advocates for the legalisation of psychedelics for spiritual purposes.

Andy Mitchell, a renegade neuroscientist who wrote *Ten Trips: The new reality of psychedelics*, also expresses concern about the prominent models for psychedelics:

> We are in danger of taking something we barely understand, something that holds huge promise for changing our perspectives—on mental health, social justice, ecological devastation and general human flourishing—and turning it into a prohibitively expensive medico-spiritual Disneyland.[3]

Mitchell points out that the model we adopt when we take psychedelics affects how we interpret the experience.

> . . . the Psychedelic Renaissance, which has to date been owned by clinical science in the West, might pupil itself in art and aesthetics—alongside history, culture and the rest of the humanities—and treat the trip not as an experiment or a therapy but as a poem, a drama, a dream . . . The convention is to separate a medical from a spiritual model, but these are commonly subdivided: medicine into neuroscientific and psychological/psychotherapeutic, spiritual into New Age or indigenous/shamanic, so that even within one broad category there are radically different ways of seeing the world, or thinking of the 'self', or understanding the meaning of a psychedelic experience . . . My experiences suggest that whatever the model, something always gets lost, neglected, simplified or confused.

One promising view of the future of psychedelics, with potential to combine the therapeutic and the spiritual, is one that mega-star MDMA researcher Rick Doblin expresses in multiple interviews as well as in a Ted Talk he gave in 2019 entitled *The Future of Psychedelic-assisted Psychotherapy:*

> We anticipate that over the next several decades, there will be thousands of psychedelic clinics established at which therapists will be able to administer MDMA, psilocybin, ketamine and other psychedelics to potentially millions of patients. These clinics can also evolve into centres where people can come for psychedelic psychotherapy, for personal growth, for couples therapy, or for spiritual, mystical experiences.[4]

In numerous interviews, Doblin points out that there are already hundreds of ketamine clinics established around the United States, for the treatment of depression, so the infrastructure, along with plenty of keen health workers, is there to offer more medicines at these clinics, as the field continues to open.

As for using psychedelics without professionals around, my LSD experience challenged me to consider cultural containers that might suit Westerners. Comparing my two LSD trips, a natural setting allowed for a superior trip—more connection to nature, more serenity. The comedown in which, for me, my body usually feels hopelessly heavy, can be a positive experience if you have a stunning view to absorb, but when I lay in bed staring at a wall, I wasted those hours, wishing them over. Yet the medical model of legalising psychedelics for mental health patients is likely to provide a clinical setting divorced from nature. How much potential is there to move clinical treatments outdoors, or even to offer views of nature through well-placed, openable windows?

One recreational psychonaut I spoke to, Paul, belongs to a regional community where friends all meet to take psychedelics—psilocybin, DMT, LSD—in the outdoors, in the fields, in the bush or on the coast. It warmed my heart when this moustachioed, heavily tattooed young man described his community:

> There's a culture of kindness. Everyone's generous and shares things—the drugs, food, knowledge, our experiences. We're all open and friendly and look out for each other. After our trips we have a great time sharing our trip reports.

Paul described how his friends tend to perceive themselves as happy refugees from modern life, especially from big cities. They reject the need to conform to society's materialist norms. Of course, it's hard to know whether psychedelics create such free spirits or if such free spirits are attracted to psychedelics. Maybe a bit of both, in a self-perpetuating cycle. Of course, this is only one of many potential psychedelic sub-cultures. I've also met experienced psychonauts who advocate for tripping alone and who want to avoid outsourcing their sovereignty to any therapist, guide or community.

I found myself conjuring a Buddhist Psychedelic Society. So many of my psychedelic experiences drew directly from Buddhist teachings, especially ayahuasca. Given the window of neuroplasticity after a psychedelic experience, I imagined using that window to attend a Buddhist retreat to practise mindfulness when my mind is at its most malleable. Not that I have the charisma, or the desire, to found a movement, but I'm happy to release the idea into the ether.

The first potential snag, however, to this brainwave is the Buddha's Fifth Precept, which requires that Buddhists avoid intoxicants. A quick google search, however, came up with the following three alternative translations of the Fifth Precept:

- Abstain from the use of intoxicating substances that cause inattention.
- Refrain from intoxicating drinks and drugs that lead to carelessness.
- Abstain from intoxicants as tending to cloud the mind.

It seems the Buddha's point is not necessarily to avoid all intoxicants but to avoid the ones that fog up the mind. The word 'psychedelic' literally means mind-revealing, or psyche-manifesting. The effect of a psychedelic, in the long run, is to clarify the state of your mind, so I'd tentatively argue that the Buddha wouldn't have a problem with them and, interestingly, most Western Buddhists I've met have tried them. Maybe it's a matter of perceiving psychedelics as sacred medicines rather than intoxicants.

Besides, the Buddha never expected Dharma practitioners to be slave-like conformists devoted to dogma. He expected us to do our own investigation to decide what is wise. I've completed an investigation into psychedelics and found them to be connectors: they connect us to ourselves, to others and to nature. With the right preparation, they increase our love for others, our self-awareness, our serenity, and for some induce an ego dissolution or 'oneness with everything'.

If the idea of a Psychedelic Buddhist Society sounds wild, consider that many thousands of Christians have already created psychedelic churches. A group originating in Brazil established the Santo Daime Church where they practise their Catholic faith, including two ayahuasca ceremonies a month. A study of over a hundred of these church members found no negative long-term effects from bi-monthly ayahuasca ceremonies. The study informs us that there are an estimated 20,000 church members practising, legally, in 23 countries including the United States, Canada and the Netherlands.[5] The Wikipedia page for Santo Daime adds Italy and France to that list.[6]

Santo Daime is not the only Christian church whose members drink ayahuasca tea in their ceremonies. União do Vegetal, translated as Union of the Plants, also originated in Brazil and boasts 21,000 members in eleven countries.[7] Their website cites a seven-year study by the Brazilian Federal Narcotics Council, which concluded:

> The followers of the sect appear to be calm and happy people. Many of them attribute family reunification, regained interest in their jobs, finding themselves and God, etc., to their religion and the tea . . . The ritual use of the tea does not appear to be disruptive or to have adverse effects upon the social interactions of the sects' followers. To the contrary, it appears to orient them towards seeking social contentment in an orderly and productive way.

Conclusion

What didn't happen

One of my original hopes for my psychedelic journey was to experience ego dissolution or ego death. On the ayahuasca trip there was the 'Sarah is Gone' scene, and on both LSD trips I felt amnesia about who I was. Still, I felt like the same old Sarah resurfaced once the trip was over, in each case. Psychonauts I've met who claim to have experienced ego death say they were never the same again and that it's a completely mind-blowing reset of everything they once assumed about life. My experiences, in retrospect, only have a dreamlike quality, and were nothing dramatic. Some would say I needed to take larger doses.

Perhaps, alternatively, the medicines are still 'cleaning me out' of material that needs releasing, before they unleash their cosmic secrets. Or maybe I should be careful what I wish for: ego death can constitute a 'spiritual emergency' for some, after which they need psychiatric intervention in order to put themselves together again. I'd nevertheless met people who raved about a completely positive experience of ego death, particularly after taking Bufo. Ironically, I'd noticed the potential for an ego death experience to be an ego-bolstering achievement to brag about on online forums.

In his article 'The Ego Doesn't Die: Why Western spirituality is so confused, and what to do about it', Alexander Beiner, who had co-facilitated my psilocybin retreat, wrote of our historically recent obsession in the West with ego death, even suggesting it might be dangerous: 'if you're looking to "erase your sense of self", what you're actually chasing is radical dissociation, and permanent psychosis'.[1]

The article continues:

> Who is the 'I' experiencing a disintegration of self? Can you become no-one, even for a moment, and still remember it? In some spiritual traditions, the answer is that it's the 'you that's everything' observing this, the 'unmoved mover' or the 'higher self'. But that is still part of your conception of self: only you are having the experience and nobody else will ever have it. The experience of 'dissolving' is inseparable from the unique point of consciousness that is located in your body, which is part of your 'sense of I'.
>
> It's more useful to talk about an 'ego-reframe' than an 'ego death'. What is happening phenomenologically in any peak mystical experience is a process of you widening your perceptual

> frame of who and what you are. For example, I might start out as 'little old me' stuck in my repetitive patterns and narrow perspectives. I then have an experience of profound connection, purpose, growth or expression. In that process, 'little old me', with all my hangups and delusions and suffering, is invited to *relate in a new way* to a reality that is both me and not me at the same time.

As with 'ego death', another experience I'd sought but hadn't encountered was that of 'becoming one with the universe', sometimes called 'unity consciousness' or 'non-duality'. I'd certainly felt the boundaries of my body dissolve on almost every trip, but nothing I'd call 'oneness with everything' despite it being a commonplace experience among psychonauts.

Another thing that didn't happen on my psychedelic journey was that, due to civil unrest, I didn't go to Peru and take ayahuasca with indigenous shamans. Fanny and Carlos, who ran the retreat in Costa Rica, were both trained by shamans, part of a lineage, but their backgrounds were those of professionals raised in Western culture. I've wondered what I missed not attending a retreat with the indigenous raised on plant wisdom, from a shamanic community. Someone who experienced an indigenous-run retreat was Englishman Jules Evans who wrote *Holiday from the Self* about his nine-day ayahuasca retreat in 2017. The shamans didn't speak English and communicated through a team of Western facilitators. Jules described a group of five shamans who interacted with him during the ayahuasca ceremonies by singing him *icaros,* which are the songs the shamans sing to people during their journeys.

> The shamans would go round the circle, each of them sitting in front of a person, assessing their psychic state, and then singing one of their *icaros*. They might blow on you or suck out some bad energy and spit it into a bowl, or anoint you with perfume, or even spit the perfume onto you . . . Maestros learn *icaros* through a process called *dieta*. They go on retreat in the jungle, fasting and consuming a particular plant, often together with ayahuasca, until eventually the spirit of that plant takes them on as a student and teaches them a song. They can then call on that spirit's help in their work, using the *icaro*. The more experienced a shaman, the more spirit-allies they have, and the more *icaros* in their shamanic juke-box.
>
> You'd receive an *icaro* from each of the five shamans over the course of the ceremony, and these were often the moments of the most intense psychedelic experience, as if the shamans really were guiding spirits into you.[2]

Through the various *icaros* that the shamans sang to Jules, he witnessed his past life as a slave-owner, he received encouragement to be more self-confident, and he reconciled with his late grandfather who had loved him despite the cold disapproval he'd displayed while alive.

One disappointment of my psychedelic journey was that the medicines didn't cure my insomnia, and, if anything, made it slightly worse. Then again, that might not be fair, as there are so many mysterious variables involved in sleep. I could still turn to the plant medicine of cannabis in the form of medicinal CBD and THC, but I wanted to avoid dependency and ultimately gave it up altogether as long-term use can become problematic.

What did I learn?

There were moments in my psychedelic journey when I vowed to make myself an expert in these fascinating medicines. Yet the more I learned about the medicines, the more mysterious they became, and the less I could make any claims, or generalisations, about them. They raise more questions than answers. No matter how much preparation you do, you won't get the trip you expected and anyone tripping next to you will have a completely different experience.

Even the researchers, the neuropsychopharmacologists, the psychiatrists and psychologists who work with the substances every day admit to bafflement about how psychedelics create the experiences they do. Not to mention that million-dollar question: did you visit a real realm, meet a real deity, receive real messages from a spirit world or was it all a projection of your subconscious mind?

Either way, each medicine taught me something.

Psilocybin helped me process, and release from my body, the vicarious trauma of my former job helping victims of sexual assault. In retrospect, it was probably ego inflation to believe, during that trip, that I was actually helping victims bear their pain. Psilocybin also helped me, through one powerful image, to forgive a character in my life I referred to as Sam, after years of trying. The psilocybin trips brought an end to my atheism and convinced me that there is a spiritual realm. I learned there was another reality, an afterlife even, and I strongly sensed other beings who I labelled at the time 'the plants'. On psilocybin, I felt the absurdity of taking life here on earth too seriously, with the exception of love, of course. Through the long afterglow, it taught me how incredibly happy I could feel for weeks on end. It re-enchanted my life.

Despite the unfathomable 'message' I received on psilocybin that Marek must embark on a psychedelic journey, Marek shows no sign of wanting to attend a psychedelic retreat and recently told me he doesn't have a good reason to risk trying psychedelics. One psychonaut I discussed this trip with suggested that I had dissociated so that Marek's childhood traumas could be processed in my body. At the time, I'd found this suggestion outrageous, but now, I'm agnostic especially after LSD gave me the impression that the traumas of historical characters were being processed in Sarah's body.

It took my plodding brain over a year to realise that maybe this trip was the result of all those years of wishing Marek and I had a common interest, some kind of shared passion. Sharing an interest in psychedelics would have filled that void. Maybe the psilocybin trip was a release of the grief of failing to connect.

I've concluded that it's best Marek stays away from psychedelics, however, as he lacks the tools that would help him benefit from the experience: an openness to therapy, a language for emotions, a spiritual framework to help make sense of his experiences or any desire for personal growth. At least, not in this lifetime. All that said, I would love, more than anything, for him to experience the simple experience of love and bliss that MDMA can give him—assuming his trip would be similar to mine. Marek said he's willing to give MDMA a try some day out of curiosity.

While my first Bufo trip remains a blur, my second led me to focus on loneliness and what small role I could play, especially with this book, to help normalise it and promote more open discussion about this inevitable experience. Bufo gave me the strength to surrender the desire for privacy on what for me has always felt like a secret, sensitive topic. Lately I've given some talks to Buddhist groups about loneliness that have been gratefully received.

Bufo cured the sciatica in my right leg (apart from a few weeks' relapse before MDMA finished the job) and taught me how releasing traumas can heal the body. The breathwork session the day after my second Bufo trip 'reactivated' the Bufo and provided me with the love of the Goddess of compassion, Kuan Yin, through a vision, and the physical sensations in my hands and arms of being held. I've often called that vision to mind when I've wanted to feel serenity, send others love, or for comfort in times of stress. I'm in a better relationship with sugar after using the window of neuroplasticity provided by Bufo, notwithstanding a serious relapse around Newtown's ice-cream shops. I now average one ice-cream a week, which is definite progress after years of daily sweet treats.

My intention for the Bufo journey had been to deal with my rejection sensitivity and the loss of friends over the COVID period following the breakdown of my marriage. While rumination and intrusive thoughts on the topic did settle down, the pain never went away and for a while I decided that psychedelics had failed me on this intention. Internal Family Systems therapy, however, which Dr Max used for my integration, showed me that I'd been trying to eradicate a part, but the part would not loosen its grip until it felt accepted, heard, comforted and fully loved up. No, the part did not respond to my attempts to murder it. I learned, however, that we can always come into a new relationship with a part. I've now stopped feeling a sense of failure when this rejection-sensitive part shows up. These days I recognise this part, comfort her, give her a cup of tea and she usually settles down. Like any part, this exile will stick around but she enjoys her new duties of helping me notice the exiled orphans in others.

I still feel weak at the knees at the very mention of MDMA, so beautiful is that memory, so beyond all my expectations. It warned me about the imminent breakup with Luke ('this one's not going to last'). It provided insight, and started a process of healing, for two exiled parts: the crying baby and tantrumming toddler within. I continue to make time to comfort these once-needy parts, usually during meditation, but also in spare moments throughout the day. MDMA granted me permission to acknowledge that some of my parts were 'broken' and gave me hope that I had the inner resources to heal myself.

Surprisingly, when it comes to cultivating self-compassion, my most influential experience may have come from the rapeh that was blown into my nose by Carlos before my first ayahuasca ceremony. For a few seconds I'd stood with my hand placed lovingly on my cheek and repeated, '*mi cariño*'. This powerful moment returns to mind often, especially during meditation. Of course, rapeh is not a psychedelic, but I remember Natasja describing it as a 'master plant teacher'.

My first two ayahuasca trips were full of messages that reside as meaningful symbols in my mind. I revisit them often as they remind me: don't get too heady and caught up in language and concepts; the Divine is within you; the Divine cares for you deeply; Luke deserves compassion; my son, Alex, carries the intergenerational trauma for the family; your shuddering is your link to the energy of other realms.

LSD emphasised the teaching that I am others and they are me: no separation. The pelican princess scene, where the nurses removed a rock of pain from my heart area, reminds me of the value in hardships and the potential for learning from them. I met my inner grumpy old lady during the second LSD trip, my irritable part with whom I was able to do valuable therapy and uncover a host of other parts. The peak hours on LSD, each time, provided an exhilarating adventure and the second trip, lying under a tree in nature, left me with a deep serenity.

My spiritual path feels especially important now. I prioritise love and learning. Meditation is something I do every day as a way to keep the lessons alive and stay connected to those other realms. I pay much more attention to my body and realise the journey has been about releasing emotional blockages from my body as much, if not more, than from my mind.

I still shudder, and shake, and make strange involuntary sounds, especially after a physical workout, when I'm tired, when I meditate or at random moments in a day, but it all magically stops when others are around.

The only other lingering 'side effect' from all my trips is tooth-grinding. I'll need to invest in an expensive mouthguard once my latest dental work settles down. If this is the only price I pay for my wondrous year of psychedelics, then I accept it.

Have psychedelics changed me? I discussed it with Dr Max.

'I have to say,' I told him, 'that I don't feel like the visions and messages I've received have shattered my reality. I need to keep working with the experiences to keep them alive in my life. Yet so many accounts of psychedelic journeys, such as most of the 54 stories in the *Mind Medicine* book, and the stories in Michael Pollan's Netflix documentary, make them sound like they changed people, once and for all, and transformed them completely. I do feel my psychedelic experiences have improved, deepened, and even re-enlivened reality for me but there's a subtlety to it. I'm still me. I know there's been healing but I can't say any of my loved ones have remarked on any difference in how I present to them.'

'I think,' Dr Max replied, 'for every person whose life has been irrevocably changed, there are another hundred who are more like you and feel they have some interesting images and messages to integrate over the years.'

I'd like to have a few months break and then continue my adventures with psychedelics into the future, maybe a couple of times a year. I'm fortunate that, for me, psychedelics have provided only fun, fascinating adventures. I've found nothing in the world more interesting to either experience or reflect back on. Like Chris Bache who took LSD 73 times, I would not advise others to do what I did. I doubt the best approach is to track down every medicine and spread yourself thinly across them all. I heard Natasja's advice more than once: settle on a medicine, stick with it, develop a relationship with it and go deep with it over time.

I particularly hope that one day I'll be able to take MDMA with someone I love but it might be a while before that happens. There's a part of me that knows I'll meet someone and it won't be too far off. Equally, there's another part of me that knows I won't. I'm not sure which part to believe.

The highlight of all my trips, particularly with MDMA and ayahuasca, echoes Alexander Beiner's conclusions about psychedelics, which he wrote about in *The Bigger Picture:*

> For me, what is most profound about the psychedelic experience is that it is an encounter with something beyond us that cares deeply about our healing; something mysterious and vast

> that loves us. For so many, it is an experience defined by an all-encompassing love and wisdom. It wants us to get better and asks nothing of us in return. This kind of love can be an inspiration, if we let it. It is the creative force that comes right from the heart of the human spirit and the universe itself. Perhaps the most radical revolution we can enact is to embody some part of this love in our day-to-day lives; in how we show up with one another; in how we treat ourselves; in how we care for the sacred land we share.[3]

I've integrated the psychedelic experience of love into my life with a daily practice of lovingkindness meditation. The medicines have taught me that cultivating a loving heart is too important, too key to it all, to neglect.

It was almost time to submit my manuscript to the publisher. On a trip to deliver his book collection to his new rental, I had a chat with Alex.

'How's the book going, Mum?'

'Okay I guess, but sometimes when I lie awake at night I feel a mini-panic, that I don't feel during the day, about revealing too much of my vulnerability.'

'But I think it's a good thing that you share your vulnerability and flaws,' he said.

'Steady there, I didn't mention any flaws,' I said.

'No, I think it's become more normal these days to talk about your vulnerabilities.'

'Really? I hope so but I feel like I've given some stand-up comedian enough material for ten years. I've written things that I've never told any living being before.'

'It'll be fine,' Alex reassured me. 'Remember, you and Dad come from a more repressed background. Especially Dad.'

I chose not to dig deeper into that statement but liked the picture he painted of a culture where people feel more free to share their emotional pain with each other. This can only ease the loneliness epidemic. One detail that had struck me reading through all the dating profiles was the number of men who chose from a list of possible interests, 'therapy', obviously feeling none of the shame that would have accompanied such an admission for a man in the pre-COVID world. An even larger number chose from that same list 'mindfulness'.

Almost every time I tell people about my psychedelic project, they ask me which medicine I liked the most, the second most and so on. I tend to cringe at this reasonable question only because I have a feeling that if I repeated my year of psychedelics, the ranking would be different. I also doubt that another person doing the same project would come up with the same ranking. For what it's worth, I provide the following ranking based on the best trip for each medicine:

First: MDMA
Second: ayahuasca
Third: psilocybin
Fourth: Bufo

Fifth: ketamine
Sixth: LSD
Seventh: mescaline

Even though I put LSD and mescaline last, I still loved my experiences and benefitted, especially from learning about Internal Family Systems therapy, in the integration. I didn't include DMT in the list, given I probably coughed out too much of it.

I'll sum up my year of psychedelics. They nudged me out of atheism into a thrilling agnosticism where anything's possible. The medicines—especially psilocybin and MDMA—made me happier than I ever remember feeling and, given the afterglow, for longer periods than I'd ever experienced, sometimes weeks. They taught me that love and learning are the priority. I feel far more connected to my fellow human, even sometimes able to see each one as 'myself'. I'm more in touch with the Divine inside me, with the Self—capital S. My meditation is deeper and connects me to the Divine within. Stretches of mindfulness, longer than any I'd experienced pre-psychedelics, happen spontaneously. I've stopped trying to murder parts of my character—the hurt parts, the irritable parts—in favour of falling in love with each part and detecting the exile that the managers and firefighters are trying to protect. My shaking and shuddering are a constant, and daily reminder of my connection to a mysterious, spirit realm.

Other than all that, I'm still just Sarah.

Turns out, she's okay.

Appendix I

Things I'd like to change about myself

1. Anxiety at night about sleep.
2. Low tolerance of frustration.
3. Irritability.
4. Prone to fixating or obsessing.
5. Impatience.
6. Crankiness when doing any form of admin.
7. Tenseness.
8. Moodiness.
9. Impatience for social occasions to end.
10. General restlessness/dissatisfaction.
11. Feeling inadequate.
12. Poor concentration.
13. Wishing I was smarter.

14. Wishing I was better looking.
15. Feeling uncared for.
16. Feeling unlikeable.
17. Longing for time alone.
18. Longing to quit my job and find something more creative.
19. Compulsions—eating sweets and Luke's chip stash, checking emails way too often.
20. Hard to feel physically comfortable in my body without lots of exercise.
21. Rejection sensitivity.
22. Insufficient community/social life.
23. Poor boundaries—absorb others' moods.
24. Missing people.
25. Loneliness.
26. Tendency to ruminate on failures and shames.
27. Living in a heightened state instead of calmly.
28. Low tolerance of stress.

Appendix 2

Inner monologue when on sugar

Gee, it's only 2 p.m. but I wouldn't mind a custard tart. Or would I prefer chocolate? Stop it! You have to at least make it to 4 p.m. Why do you always do this to yourself? You know eating sweets only makes you feel queasy and lethargic, like yesterday. You promised you wouldn't do it again—when are you going to stop? Oh, but that initial sugar rush is a real pick-me-up and I crave it sooo bad. Maybe an ice-cream would hit the spot better. One of these days I'll give up and won't have my day dominated by cravings and the mental merry-go-round of: Should I? Shouldn't I?

I just need a lift—I feel a bit dull and lacking in energy. Sugar at least gives me an energy injection. But don't forget the crash later—and the regret. That's it. No sugar today. Oh, but I want it so bad. Tough! Oh no, what am I doing? I seem to be in the lift down to the convenience store and it's only 3.30. Why can't I control my own actions? I didn't even realise I was walking to the lift—I just kept visualising that chocolate bar and now, here I am. In the lift. It's so embarrassing, that shopkeeper must think I'm pathetic coming every day for my hit. The walk of shame to the chocolate shelf.

[Gobble the chocolate at my desk hoping nobody interrupts my one minute of bliss.]

[Later] Why did I do that? It's not sitting well in my stomach and I've ruined my appetite for dinner. I must do better tomorrow. I need to quit altogether but can't seem to get through a day without it. Do I have to punish myself again by watching anti-sugar documentaries or reading anti-sugar books? They do seem to work for a while but there are things I'd rather do with my time than re-educate myself, for the umpteenth time, about the harms of sugar. I wish I could control it. Maybe I need a new approach . . . like one treat a week? Or a food diary to keep me accountable.

Acknowledgements

ENORMOUS THANKS TO MEDICINE Woman and Wisdom Keeper Natasja Pelgrom and to *curanderos* Carlos and Fanny in Costa Rica. To my MDMA guide 'Sasha' and my integration therapist Dr 'Max' as well as Holotropic Breathwork guide Lynsey Chan.

I give thanks for generously granting me permission to quote from your work to: Alexander Beiner, Dr Rick Strassman, Professor David Nutt, *The Conversation*, Nick and Jimmy at Psychedelic Passage, Jules Evans, Simone Dowding and Graeme Sudholz, and huge thanks to Christopher M. Bache who's done so much of the heavy lifting in the psychedelic space. Further thanks for allowing me to quote from your personal stories to: Trish, Marek, 'Jimmy', Mike, Elmer, Sam, Ter and Darren.

Editors Samantha Kent and Melissa-Jane Fogarty provided insightful edits that greatly enhanced the book and Annette Barlow showed most generous faith in the project. Gratitude also to Tom Flood and Anne Reilly for some astute early advice on the manuscript.

Hearty love to Zac, Alex, each of their very special girlfriends, Mum and all the patient friends who have listened and supported.

Notes

Introduction

1 R.R. Griffiths, W.A. Richards, U. McCann, and R. Jesse, 'Psilocybin can occasion mystical-type experiences having substantial and sustained personal meaning and spiritual significance', *Psychopharmacology*, 2006, p. 9, DOI: 10.1007/s00213-006-0457-5.

2 J. Markoff, *What the Dormouse Said: How the 60s counterculture shaped the personal computer industry*, Viking Penguin: New York, 2005.

3 M. Pollan, *How To Change Your Mind: The new science of psychedelics*, Penguin Books: United Kingdom, 2018, p. 7.

4 A. Isaacson, 'Return of the Fungi', Mother Jones, 2009, <www.motherjones.com/environment/2009/11/paul-stamets-mushroom/>, (17 January, 2024).

5 B. Carey, 'Tim Ferriss, the Man Who Put His Money Behind Psychedelic Medicine', *The New York Times,* 2019, <www.nytimes.com/2019/09/06/health/ferriss-psychedelic-drugs-depression.html>, (24 October 2023).

6 C. Ly, A.C. Greb, L.P. Cameron, J.M. Wong, E.V. Barragan, P.C. Wilson, K.F. Burbach, S.S. Zarandi, A. Sood, M.R. Paddy, W.C. Duim, M.Y. Dennis, A.K. McAllister, K.M. Ori-McKenney, J.A. Gray, and

D.E. Olson, 'Psychedelics Promote Structural and Functional Neural Plasticity', *PubMed Central*, 2018, <www.ncbi.nlm.nih.gov/pmc/articles/PMC6082376/>, (24 October 2023), DOI: 10.1016/j.celrep.2018.05.022.

7 R. Millière, R.L. Carhart-Harris, L. Roseman, F-M Trautwein, and A. Berkovich-Ohana, 'Psychedelics, Meditation, and Self-Consciousness', *Frontiers in Psychology*, 2018, vol. 9, <www.frontiersin.org/articles/10.3389/fpsyg.2018.01475/full>, (24 October 2023).

8 D. Harris, (Host), (2015–present), podcast 'Psychedelics and Meditation–Michael Pollan', September 2021, *Ten Percent Happier* [Audio podcast] Spotify, <https://open.spotify.com/episode/10oOyE1KhRmFh28gkO1CM3>, (25 October 2023).

Chapter 1: Isn't it all a bit risky?

1 D.J. Nutt, L.A. King, L.D. Philips on behalf of the Independent Scientific Committee on Drugs, 'Drug harms in the UK: a multicriteria decision analysis', *The Lancet*, Volume 376, Issue 9752 (2010), pp. 1558–65.

2 J. Rogan, (Host), (2009–present), podcast '#1661—Rick Doblin', 5 June 2021, *The Joe Rogan Experience* [Video podcast], Spotify, <https://open.spotify.com/episode/1Z8lzhvHCMv0c8qZWXbzK>, (25 October 2023), (2 hours 8 mins).

3 J. Fadiman, *The Psychedelic Explorer's Guide: Safe, therapeutic, and sacred journeys*, Park Street Press: Rochester, Vermont, 2011.

4 M. Szalavitz, 'Aaron Alexis and the Dark Side of Meditation', *TIME USA*, 2013, <www.healthland.time.com/2013/09/17/aaron-alexis-and-the-dark-side-of-meditation/>, (25 October 2023).

5 D. Nutt, *Psychedelics: The revolutionary drugs that could change your life—a guide from the expert*, Yellow Kite: London, 2023, pp. 275, 280–1.

6 T. Trimingham, *Not My Family, Never My Child: What to do if someone you love is a drug user*, Allen & Unwin: Sydney, 2009.

7 Telephone number for Family Drug Support: 1300 368 186 (24 hours), <www.fds.org.au>.

8 A.K. Schlag, 'Percentages of problem drug use and their implications for policy making: A review of the literature', *Sage Journals: Drug Science, Policy and Law*, 2020, <https://journals.sagepub.com/doi.org/10.1177/2050324520904540>, (25 October 2023).

9 P. Hayes, 'Many people use drugs—but here's why most don't become addicts', *The Conversation*, 2015, <https://theconversation.com/many-people-use-drugs-but-heres-why-most-dont-become-addicts-35504>, (27 September 2024).

10 The exceptions are Australian Capital Territory and, as of 2023, Queensland.

11 Anonymous, *Go Ask Alice*, Prentice Hall: New York, 1971.

12 R. Emerson, *Unmask Alice: LSD, satanic panic, and the imposter behind the world's most notorious diaries*, BenBella Books: Dallas, Texas, 2022.

13 J. Evans, *Holiday from the Self: An accidental ayahuasca adventure*, self-published, available from Amazon, 2019.

14 J. Evans, O. Robinson, E.K. Argyri, S. Suseelan, A. Murphy-Beiner and R. McAlpine, 'Extended Difficulties Following the Use of Psychedelic Drugs: A Mixed Methods Study', *SSRN*, June 21, 2023, <https://ssrn.com/abstract=4505228 or http://dx.doi.org/10.2139/ssrn.4505228>, (27 September 2024).

Chapter 2: Lead-up to my first retreat

1 B. van der Kolk, *The Body Keeps the Score: Mind, brain and body in the transformation of trauma*, Penguin Books: United Kingdom, 2015.

Chapter 3: Psilocybin in the Netherlands

1 'French Tourist in Amsterdam Commits Suicide After Using "Magic Mushrooms"', *Simply Amsterdam*, 27 March 2007, <www.simplyamsterdam.nl/news_detail.php?a=French_tourist_in_Amsterdam_commits_suicide_after_using_magic_mushrooms>, (25 October 2023).

2 R.P.J. Koning, A. Benschop, C. Wijffels, and J. Noijen, 'Visitors of the Dutch drug checking services: Profile and drug use experience', *International Journal of Drug Policy*, vol. 95, September 2021, <www.sciencedirect.com/science/article/abs/pii/S0955395921001997>, (25 October 2023), DOI: 10.1016/j.drugpo.2021.103293.

3 G. Roberts, 'What has Canberra's fixed-site pill and drug testing clinic found in its first month?', *ABC News*, 2022, <www.abc.net.au/news/2022-

08-25/act-pill-drug-testing-results-revealed-mdma-heroin/101371644>, (23 January, 2024).

Chapter 4: Second psilocybin ceremony

1 Index (Front Page): Erowid Experience Vaults. <www.erowid.org/experiences/>, (27 September 2024).

Chapter 5: Lead-up to Bufo in Portugal

1 C. Hughes, and A. Stevens, 'The Effects of Decriminalization of Drug Use in Portugal', *The Beckley Foundation Drug Policy Programme*, 2007, briefing paper 14, <https://beckleyfoundation.org/wp-content/uploads/2016/04/paper_14.pdf>, (25 October 2023).
2 ThirdWave, 'The Ultimate Guide to 5-MeO-DMT', 2024, <https://thethirdwave.co/psychedelics/5-meo-dmt/>, (11 January 2024).
3 P. McConnell, 'Decoding the Difference Between 5-MeO-DMT and N, N-DMT', *Microdose*, 2022, <https://microdose.buzz/news/decoding-the-difference-between-5-MeO-DMT-and-N-N-DMT/>, (25 October 2023).
4 A.K. Davis, S. So, R.L. Lancelotta, J. Barsuglia, and R.R. Griffiths, '5-methoxy-N, N-dimethyltryptamine (5-MeO-DMT) used in a naturalistic group setting is associated with unintended improvements in depression and anxiety', *The American Journal of Drug and Alcohol Abuse*, 2019, pp. 161–69, DOI: 10.1080/00952990.2018.1545024.
5 '5-MeO-DMT (Bufo)', Drug Science, <www.drugscience.org.uk/drug-information/5-meo-dmt/#5MeODMT4>, (12 January 2024).
6 A. Most, *The Psychedelic Toad of the Sonoran Desert*, Arizona, 1983, <www.erowid.org/archive/sonoran_desert_toad/almost.htm>, (25 October 2023).
7 N. Pelgrom, 'The Deep Dive into *Bufo alvarius* (5-MeO-DMT)', in T. Read, and M. Papaspyrou, (ed.), *Psychedelics and Psychotherapy: The healing potential of expanded states*, Park Street Press: Rochester, Vermont, 2021, Chapter 17.
8 The freedom tribe (the-freedom-tribe.com), <www.the-freedom-tribe.com> (27 September 2024).
9 M. Sampayo, 'French Influence on Portuguese Architects in the Age of Enlightenment', *IOP Conference Series*, 2017, <https://iopscience.iop.org/

article/10.1088/1757-899X/245/5/052059>, (25 October 2023), DOI: 10.1088/1757-899X/245/5/052059.

Chapter 8: Reflecting on the Bufo retreat

1 A.M.O. Bernal, C.L. Raison, R.L. Lancelotta, and A.K. Davis, 'Reactivations after 5-methoxy-N,N-dimethyltryptamine use in naturalistic settings: An initial exploratory analysis of the phenomenon's predictors and its emotional valence', *Frontiers in Psychiatry*, 2022, <https://doi.org/10.3389/fpsyt.2022.1049643>, (25 October 2023).

2 M. Pollan, *This Is Your Mind on plants: Opium-caffeine-mescaline*, Penguin: United Kingdom, 2021, p. 214.

Chapter 9: Holotropic Breathwork in Sydney

1 S. & C. Grof, *Holotropic Breathwork: A new approach to self-exploration and therapy*, SUNY Press: New York, 2010, p. 30.

2 Psilocybin and MDMA for treatment-resistant depression and PTSD, respectively, would be legalised as medicines in Australia on 1 July 2023. Mind Medicine Australia (see chapter 21) has established a fund to help finance psychedelic-assisted psychotherapy.

3 S. & C. Grof, *Holotropic Breathwork*, p. xiv.

4 T. Miller, and L. Nielsen, 'Measure of Significance of Holotropic Breathwork in the Development of Self-Awareness', *The Journal of Alternative and Complementary Medicine*, 2015, vol. 21, no. 12, pp. 796–803, <https://pubmed.ncbi.nlm.nih.gov/26565611>, (25 October 2023), DOI: 10.1089/acm.2014.0297.

5 J. Eyerman, 'A Clinical Report of Holotropic Breathwork in 11,000 Psychiatric Inpatients in a Community Hospital Setting', *Psychedelics in Psychology and Psychiatry*, Spring 2013, vol. 23, no.1, <https://maps.org/news/bulletin/a-clinical-report-of-holotropic-breathwork-in-11000-psychiatric-inpatients-in-a-community-hospital-setting/>, (October 25 2023).

6 S. & C. Grof, *Holotropic Breathwork*, p.12.

7 S. & C. Grof, p. xiv.

8 S. & C. Grof, p. 55.

Chapter 10: Lead-up to MDMA in Australia

1. J. Rogan, (Host), (2009–present), podcast '#1661—Rick Doblin', 5 June 2021, *The Joe Rogan Experience* [Video podcast], Spotify, <https://open.spotify.com/episode/1Z8lzhvHCMv0c8qZWXbzK>, (25 October 2023), (12 minutes 15 seconds).
2. H. Devlin, 'The undersea and the ecstasy: MDMA leaves octopuses loved up', *The Guardian Australia*, 2018, <www.theguardian.com/science/2018/sep/20/mdma-makes-octopuses-more-sociable>, (25 October 2023).
3. J. Healy, and C. Sibthorpe, 'Groovin the Moo pill tests find lethal stimulant, paint and toothpaste in drugs', *ABC Radio Canberra*, 2018, <www.abc.net.au/news/2018-04-30/groovin-the-moo-pill-testing-finds-lethal-product/9710112>, (25 October 2023).
4. G. Roberts, 'What has Canberra's fixed-site pill and drug testing clinic found in its first month?', *ABC News*, 2022, <www.abc.net.au/news/2022-08-25/act-pill-drug-testing-results-revealed-mdma-heroin/101371644s>, (23 January, 2024).
5. A. Roxburgh, J. Lappin, 'MDMA-related deaths in Australia 2000 to 2018', *International Journal of Drug Policy*, 2020, vol. 76, <www.sciencedirect.com/science/article/abs/pii/S0955395919303445>, (18 January, 2024).
6. Six-hundred thousand Australians use MDMA each year according to The National Drug Strategy Household Survey 2019. For all MDMA, on its own or with other drugs, let's divide the 392 deaths over 18 years by 18 to get yearly deaths of 22. Yearly deaths of 22 divided by the 600,000 annual MDMA users is 0.00004. For MDMA on its own, 55 deaths in 18 years translates to a yearly rate of 3 deaths. Divide that by the 600,000 users and you get 0.000008.
7. 'International Road Safety Comparisons—Annual', The Department of Infrastructure, Transport, Regional Development, Communications and the Arts, 2022, <www.bitre.gov.au/publications/ongoing/international_road_safety_comparisons>, (25 October 2023).
8. 'Prof David Nutt sacked from Advisory Council on the Misuse of Drugs', Institute of Alcohol Studies, 2009, <www.ias.org.uk/news/prof-david-nutt-sacked-from-advisory-council-on-the-misuse-of-drugs>, (25 October 2023).
9. R. Strassman, M.D., *The Psychedelic Handbook: A practical guide to psilocybin, LSD, ketamine, MDMA, and DMT/ayahuasca*, Ulysses Press: Berkeley, California, 2022.
10. R. Strassman, M.D., *The Psychedelic Handbook*, chapter 8.

11 J. Nguyen, N. Levich, (Hosts), (2022–present), podcast 'How Psychedelics Help Release Traumatic Residue', [Video podcast], <www.psychedelicpassage.com/how-psychedelics-help-release-traumatic-residue/>, (26 October 2023).

12 'There is suffering' is a common but lazy translation of the First Noble truth that might more accurately be translated as something like, 'Everything is marked by unsatisfactoriness due to the impermanence of anything we want to grasp onto'.

13 'Alcohol, tobacco & other drugs in Australia, Harm minimisation', Australian Institute of Health and Welfare, 2023, <www.aihw.gov.au/reports/alcohol/alcohol-tobacco-other-drugs-australia/contents/harm-minimisation>, (26 October 2023).

Chapter 11: MDMA in Queensland

1 A. Waldman, *A Really Good Day: How microdosing made a mega difference in my mood, my marriage, and my life*, Knopf: New York, 2017.

2 A. Waldman, 'Truly, Madly, Guiltily', *The New York Times*, 2005, <www.nytimes.com/2005/03/27/fashion/truly-madly-guiltily.html>, (25 October 2023).

Chapter 12: Lead-up to ayahuasca in Costa Rica

1 C.S. Grob, 'The Psychology of Ayahuasca', Chapter 2 in R. Metzner (ed.), *The Ayahuasca Experience: A sourcebook on the sacred vine of spirits*, Park Street Press: Rochester, Vermont, 2014.

2 R. Metzner (ed.), *The Ayahuasca Experience,* Introduction.

3 'Costa Rica', Happy Planet Index, Hot or Cool Institute gGmbH, <https://happyplanetindex.org/countries/?c=CRI>, (26 October 2023).

4 J. Bremner, A. Harrell, B. Kluepfel, and M. Vorhees, *Lonely Planet Costa Rica*, 14th Edition, Lonely Planet Global Limited, 2022.

5 M.B. Sheridan, 'Costa Rica, laid-back land of "pura vida," succumbing to drug violence', *The Washington Post*, 2023, <www.washingtonpost.com/world/2023/03/22/costa-rica-violence-crime-drugs>, (25 October 2023).

6 'About drug law reform in Costa Rica', UN Drug Control: Drug Law Reform, 2016, <www.tni.org/en/publication/about-drug-law-reform-in-costa-rica>, (26 October 2023).
7 C. Jimenez, 'Best Ayahuasca Retreat-Costa Rica Reviews', *Pura Vida Moms*, 2022, <www.puravidamoms.com/ayahuasca-costa-rica/>, (26 October 2023).

Chapter 13: First ayahuasca ceremony

1 S. & C. Grof, *Holotropic Breathwork: A new approach to self-exploration and therapy*, SUNY Press: New York, 2010, pp. 24 and 132.

Chapter 14: Second ayahuasca ceremony

1 J. Kornfield, *After the Ecstasy, the Laundry: How the heart grows wise on the spiritual path*, Bantam Books: London, 2000.

Chapter 15: Third ayahuasca ceremony

1 Dr C.M. Bache, *LSD and the Mind of the Universe: Diamonds from Heaven*, Park Street Press: Rochester, Vermont, 2019, pp. 205–6.

Chapter 16: Lead-up to LSD in Sydney

1 Yes, I'd had a boyfriend between Marek and Luke. Don't ask.
2 D. Schreiber, *Alone*, Reaktion Books: London, 2023, pp. 57–58, 62, 109, (Translated from German by Ben Fergusson).
3 Sarvananda, *Solitude and Loneliness: A Buddhist view*, Windhorse Publications: Cambridge, United Kingdom, 2012, pp. 10, 27, 31.
4 *How To Change Your Mind*, Netflix, Directed by L. Walker and A. Ellwood, Executive Producer A. Gibney, Creator J. Adler, Jigsaw Productions in association with Tree Tree Tree, Episode 1, <Watch How To Change Your Mind | Netflix Official Site>, <www.netflix.com/au/title/80229847>, (18 January, 2024).

5 W. Thoricatha, 'The Building Blocks of Life: Kary Mullis and Francis Crick's Psychedelic Breakthrough', *Psychedelic Times*, 2015, <https://psychedelictimes.com/building-blocks-life-karry-mullis-francis-crick-psychedelic-breakthrough>, (12 January, 2024).

6 Dr C.M. Bache, *LSD and the Mind of the Universe: Diamonds from Heaven*, Park Street Press: Rochester, Vermont, 2019, pp. 4, 51, 99, 218–19, 225–6.

7 Bache spent three years exploring his former lives through hypnotherapy 'becoming intimately familiar with about a dozen of them'. He presented the empirical evidence for reincarnation in his first book, *Lifecycles* (1990).

8 R.C. Schwartz, and M. Sweezy, *Internal Family Systems Therapy: Second Edition*, Guilford Press: New York, 2020, pp. 32–6.

9 R.C. Schwartz, and M. Sweezy, *Internal Family Systems Therapy*, pp. 257–8, 276.

Chapter 17: LSD in Sydney

1 Microdoses of psilocybin tend to be ten per cent of a standard dose, taken several times a week. The effects are 'imperceptible' but can ease anxiety and depression and, in some cases, physical pain, although the latter impact has not been sufficiently researched to date. G. Conroy, 'Can microdosing psychedelics improve your mental health? Here's what the science says', *ABC News* online, 2022,<www.abc.net.au/news/health/2022-07-03/mental-health-microdosing-psychedelics-magic-mushrooms/101154616>, (5 February, 2024).

2 C. Muscara, 'Corey Muscara's Post' LinkedIn, <www.linkedin.com/posts/corymuscara_heres-a-provocative-statement-if-you-want-activity-6987518390638698496-p5rX>, (12 January, 2024).

Chapter 19: DMT near Newcastle

1 *How To Change Your Mind*, Netflix, Directed by L. Walker and A. Ellwood, Executive Producer A. Gibney, Creator J. Adler, Jigsaw Productions in association with Tree Tree Tree, Episode 2, < Watch How To Change Your Mind | Netflix Official Site>, <www.netflix.com/au/title/80229847>, (18 January 2024).

2 ThirdWave, 'The Ultimate Guide to 5-MeO-DMT', 2024, <5-MeO-DMT Guide: 5-MeO Experience, Benefits, & Effects – Third Wave (thethirdwave.co)>, (11 January, 2024).

3 V. Cakic, J. Potkonyak, and A. Marshall, 'Dimethyltryptamine (DMT): subjective effects and patterns of use among Australian recreational users', *Drug and Alcohol Dependence*, vol. 111, Issues 1–2, 1 September 2010, pp. 30–37.

4 A.K. Davis, J.M. Clifton, E.G. Weaver, E.S. Hurwitz, M.W. Johnson, and R.R. Griffiths, 'Survey of entity encounter experiences occasioned by inhaled N,N-dimethyltryptamine: Phenomenology, interpretation, and enduring effects', vol. 34, Issue 9, 2020, <https://pubmed.ncbi.nlm.nih.gov/32345112/>, (25 October, 2023).

5 J. Dean, 'Drug session showed me "huge vision of God", reveals Paul McCartney', *The Sunday Times*, 2018, <www.thetimes.co.uk/article/drug-session-showed-me-huge-vision-of-god-reveals-paul-mccartney-2s9p8kg5m>, (25 October 2023).

6 R. Strassman, M.D., *DMT: The Spirit Molecule: A doctor's revolutionary research into the biology of near-death and mystical experiences*, Park Street Press: Rochester, Vermont, 2000.

7 E.W. Dolan, 'New study offers a detailed glimpse into the otherworldly encounters produced by the psychedelic drug DMT', *Psychedelic Drugs,* 2022, 'Psychedelics can alter a person's core metaphysical beliefs for as long as six months after use, study suggests', <www.psypost.org/psychedelics-can-alter-a-persons-core-metaphysical-beliefs-for-as-long-as-six-months-after-use-study-suggests/>, (3 January, 2024).

Chapter 20: Mescaline and ketamine in Sydney

1 A. Huxley, *The Doors of Perception*, Harper and Row: New York, 1954.

2 M. Jay, *Mescaline: A global history of the first psychedelic*, Yale University Press: London, 2019.

3 D. Nutt, *Psychedelics: The revolutionary drugs that could change your life–a guide from the expert*, Yellow Kite: London, 2023, p. 110.

4 R. Robison, 'Lessons learned from 10,000 doses of ketamine with Dr Reid Robison', Mind Medicine Australia, <www.youtube.com/watch?v=UbFviHeX-hk >, (22 January, 2024).

5 R. Nardou, E. Sawyer, Y. J. Song, M. Wilkinson, Y. Padovan-Hernandez, J.L. de Deus, N. Wright, C. Lama, S. Faltin, L.A. Goff, G.L. Stein-O'Brien,

and G. Dölen, 'Psychedelics reopen the social reward learning critical period', *Nature*, 2023, <https://irp.cdn-website.com/b0dc26db/files/uploaded/published%20Nardou%20et%20al%202023%20NATURE.pdf>, (22 January, 2024).

6 R. Strassman, M.D., *The Psychedelic Handbook: A practical guide to psilocybin, LSD, ketamine, MDMA, and DMT/ayahuasca*, Ulysses Press: Berkeley, California, 2022.

7 Alcohol and Drug Foundation, 'Ketamine use in Australia', 2022, <https://adf.org.au/insights/ketamine-use-australia/>, (22 January, 2024).

Chapter 21: Psychedelic-assisted psychotherapy

1 *How To Change Your Mind*, Netflix, Directed by L. Walker and A. Ellwood, Executive Producer A. Gibney, Creator J. Adler, Jigsaw Productions in association with Tree Tree Tree, Episode 1, <Watch How To Change Your Mind | Netflix Official Site>, <www.netflix.com/au/title/80229847>, (18 January, 2024).

2 Blossom Analysis <https://blossomanalysis.com/clinical-trials/>, (18 January, 2024).

3 Number of trials: psilocybin (eighteen), MDMA (ten), LSD (three, all in New Zealand), Ibogaine (three, all in New Zealand), DMT (two), Iprocin (one) and ayahuasca (one). 'Clinical Trials', Mind Medicine Australia, 2024, <https://mindmedicineaustralia.org.au/clinical-trials>, (18 January, 2024).

4 R. Griffiths, M. Johnson, M. Carducci, A. Umbricht, W. Richards, B. Richards, M. Cosimano, and M. Klinedinst, 'Psilocybin produces substantial and sustained decreases in depression and anxiety in patients with life-threatening cancer: A randomized double-blind trial', *Journal of Psychopharmacology*, 2016, <https://pubmed.ncbi.nlm.nih.gov/27909165/>, (18 January, 2024).

5 Tania adds an exception: 'While every suffering person should have the right to safe and effective treatments, at this stage in the research, until the impacts are better understood, people with psychotic disorders such as bipolar, schizophrenia and various personality disorders are not eligible for treatment with psychedelics. The field is advancing very rapidly, and many researchers are interested in the potential of psychedelic-assisted therapies to treat these and a range of other conditions.'

Chapter 22: The future of psychedelics

1 A. Beiner, *The Bigger Picture: How psychedelics can help us make sense of the world*, Hay House: London, 2023, p. xix.

2 Dr C.M. Bache, *LSD and the Mind of the Universe: Diamonds from Heaven*, Park Street Press: Rochester, Vermont, 2019.

3 A. Mitchell, *Ten Trips: The new reality of psychedelics*, The Bodley Head: London, 2023, pp. 310, 298, 303.

4 R. Doblin, 'The future of psychedelic-assisted psychotherapy', TED Talk, YouTube <www.bing.com/videos/riverview/relatedvideo?q=%22Rick%20Doblin%22%20%22Ketamine%20clinics%22%20future%20of%20psychedelics&mid=6ACB559933678C103C416ACB559933678C103C41&ajaxhist=0, (20 December 2023).

5 J.C. Bouso, D. González, S. Fondevila, M. Cutchet, X. Fernández, P.C.R. Barbosa, M.A. Alcázar-Córcoles, W.S. Araújo, M.J. Barbanoj, J.M. Fábregas, and J. Riba, 'Personality, Psychopathology, Life Attitudes and Neuropsychological Performance among Ritual Users of Ayahuasca: A longitudinal study', *National Library of Medicine*, <www.ncbi.nlm.nih.gov/pmc/articles/PMC3414465/>, <https://en.wikipedia.org/wiki/Santo_Daime>, (19 December 2023).

6 <https://en.wikipedia.org/wiki/Santo_Daime>, (11 January 2024).

7 Centro Espírita Beneficente União do Vegetal in the United States, <https://udvusa.org>, (19 December 2023).

Conclusion

1 A. Beiner, 'The Ego Doesn't Die: Why Western spirituality is so confused, and what to do about it: Ego-death and the science of transformation', The Bigger Picture Substack, 2023, <https://beiner.substack.com/p/the-ego-doesnt-die-why-western-spirituality>, (5 December 2023).

2 J. Evans, *Holiday from the Self: An accidental ayahuasca adventure*, self-published, available from Amazon, 2019, p.18.

3 A. Beiner, *The Bigger Picture: How psychedelics can help us make sense of the world*, Hay House: London, 2023, pp. xix, 232–3.

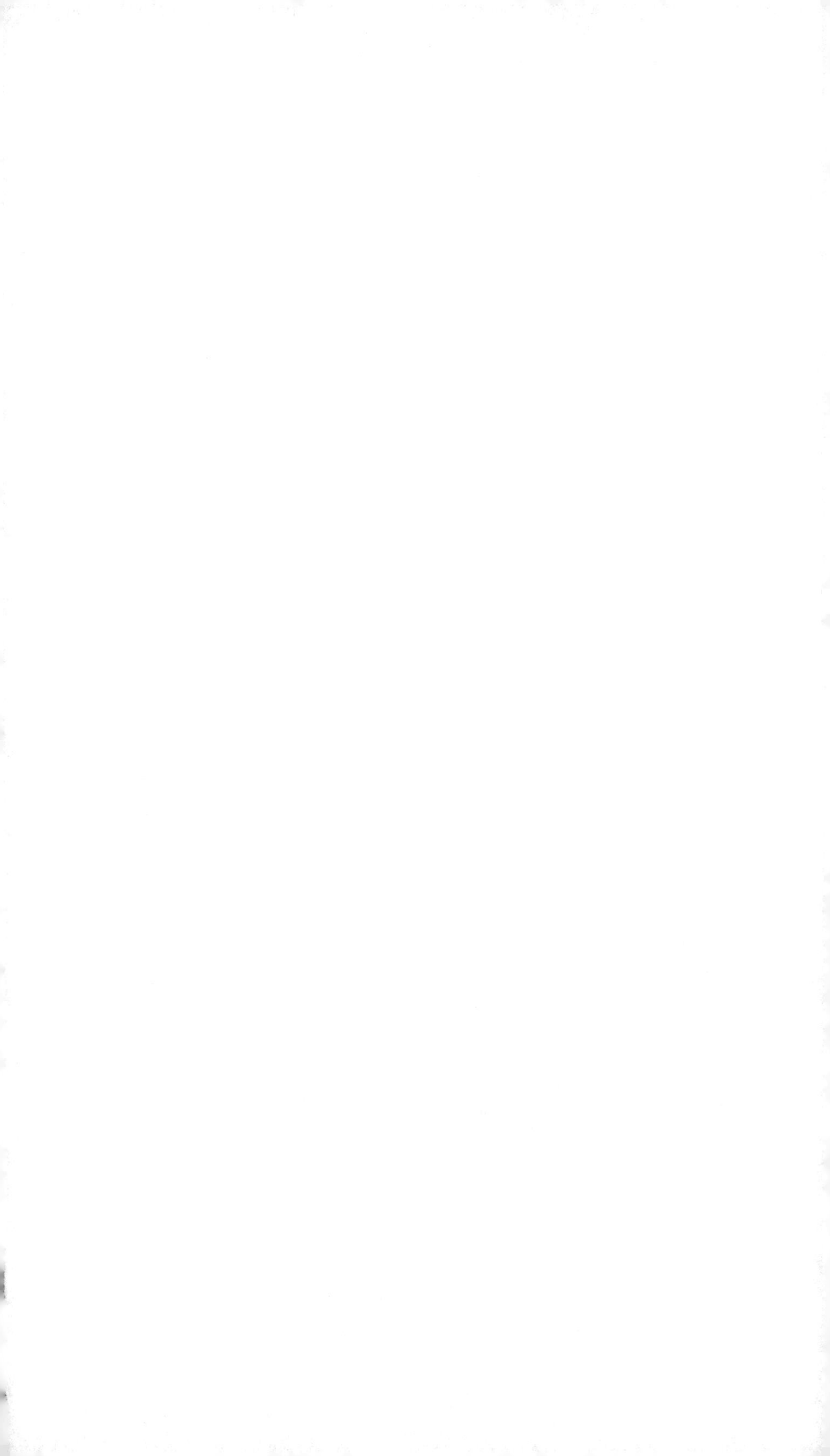